Contents

Helicobacter pylori

A. W. HARRIS MD MRCP

& J. J. MISIEWICZ BSc MB FRCP

Both of Department of Gastroenterology & Nutrition
Central Middlesex Hospital NHS Trust
Acton Lane, Park Royal, London NW10 7NS, UK

Blackwell
Healthcare
Communications

Provided as a
service to medicine by

Wyeth

© 1996 by
Blackwell Healthcare
Communications Ltd
1 University House, Ealing Green
London W5 5EA
An imprint of
Blackwell Science Ltd
Editorial Offices:
Osney Mead, Oxford OX2 0EL
25 John Street, London WCIN 2BL
23 Ainslie Place, Edinburgh EH3 6AJ
238 Main Street, Cambridge
    Massachusetts 02142, USA
54 University Street, Carlton
    Victoria 3053, Australia

Other Editorial Offices:
Arnette Blackwell SA
    224, Boulevard Saint Germain
    75007 Paris, France

Blackwell Wissenschafts-Verlag GmbH
    Kurfürstendamm 57
    10707 Berlin, Germany

    Zehetnergasse 6
    A-1140 Wien
    Austria

First published 1996

Set by Excel Typesetters Co., Hong Kong
Printed and bound in Great Britain
at the Alden Press Limited,
Oxford and Northampton

The Blackwell Healthcare
Communications logo is a trade mark
of Blackwell Science Ltd,
registered at the United Kingdom
Trade Marks Registry

DISTRIBUTORS

    Marston Book Services Ltd
    PO Box 269
    Abingdon
    Oxon OX14 4YN
    (*Orders*: Tel: 01235 465500
                Fax: 01235 465555)

USA
    Blackwell Science, Inc.
    238 Main Street
    Cambridge, MA 02142
    (*Orders*: Tel: 800 215-1000
                617 876-7000
                Fax: 617 492-5263)

Canada
    Copp Clark Professional
    200 Adelaide Street West, 3rd Floor
    Toronto, Ontario
    Canada M5H 1W7
    (*Orders*: Tel: 416-597-1616
                800-815-9417
                Fax: 416-597-1617)

Australia
    Blackwell Science Pty Ltd
    54 University Street
    Carlton, Victoria 3053
    (*Orders*: Tel: 03 9347 0300
                Fax: 03 9349 3016)

Catalogue records for this title
are available from the British Library and
the Library of Congress

ISBN 0-86542-639-2

Foreword

The standard therapy for a peptic ulcer when I was a medical student was an antacid, possibly combined with carbenoxolone. Patients with intractable ulcers were occasionally admitted to a medical ward 'for intensive therapy' and senior consultants sometimes considered wistfully whether it would be appropriate to revisit the 'milk drip'. As a registrar I was involved in the early studies with H_2-receptor antagonists, which many of us believed at the time were going to be unsurpassable remedies in the treatment of peptic ulceration and gastro-oesophageal reflux. Two major developments, however, soon followed, namely the discovery of *Helicobacter pylori* and the characterisation of the proton pump and the production of drugs which inhibit its action. The idea that peptic ulcer, gastritis and gastric cancer could be due to a single infectious disease was in those early days totally untenable. We now know differently, the discovery of this organism has turned the science and clinical practice of these gastro-duodenal diseases on its head.

This succinct, focused text by Adam Harris and George Misiewicz summarises most of what we know about the molecular pathogenesis, clinical manifestations and current approaches to the management of this infection. The book is clearly written and appropriately illustrated with figures and diagrams and further enhanced by summary statements and key points in the margins. The book is aimed at general practitioners but I suspect it will have a wider appeal; an ideal starting point for medical students, trainees in gastroenterology and other medical specialists, and possibly for some of those senior consultants who still just about remember 'the milk drip'.

There are a number of controversial issues in the world of *H. pylori*, one of which is 'who should be treated?' The authors take an appropriately conservative view and recommend that prescribing eradication therapy should be restricted to currently published guidelines. However, those of us in clinical practice, both in hospitals and the community, know that parents are extremely well informed about this infection and are asking for treatment irrespective of whether their own particular problem falls within the current guidelines. I have a sneaking suspicion that it will not to be too long before self-testing and self therapy is the order of the day!

Michael J.G. Farthing
Professor of Gastroenterology
September 1996

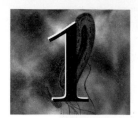

Introduction

The discovery of *H. pylori* (Fig. 1.1) has opened new opportunities in the management of upper gastrointestinal (GI) disorders, with the cure for chronic ulcer disease being possible for the first time. In fact, such indications for eradication therapy that have been firmly established remain quite limited. These indications are still those proposed by the National Institutes of Health (NIH) some 3 years ago, namely only patients with *H. pylori*-positive duodenal (DU) or gastric (GU) ulcers should be offered eradication therapy. This general precept holds good, but can be modified in the light of clinical experience.

All newly diagnosed DU patients and those on maintenance therapy with acid-suppressive agents should be offered *H. pylori* eradication therapy

Firmly diagnosed patients with DU do not need any further tests; if they are not consuming ulcerogenic drugs their ulcers can be assumed to be *H. pylori*-related and eradication therapy should be offered. All newly diagnosed DUs should be offered anti-*H. pylori* treatment at the time of diagnosis; there is no need for an initial trial of acid suppressive therapy. An endoscopic diagnosis is preferable, but suggestive barium meal appearances coupled with a positive *H. pylori* serology are enough evidence for treatment. The presence of duodenitis in an *H. pylori*-positive patient is an indication for treatment, and so is acid-suppressive maintenance therapy for peptic ulcer. It is arguable that confirmation of successful eradication may not be necessary — preliminary studies suggest close correspondence between eradication and remission of symptoms.

All GUs need endoscopic evaluation to confirm the absence of cancer and to establish *H. pylori* status. All *H. pylori*-positive GUs merit eradication treatment.

At present, there is no firm evidence of significant benefit from *H. pylori* eradication in NUD

At present, firm evidence of any significant benefit from eradication of *H. pylori* in non-ulcer dyspepsia (NUD) (functional dyspepsia, ulcer type) is lacking. Many clinicians hold the view that indiscriminate treatment of all *H. pylori*-positive dyspeptics who have no ulcer, or duodenitis, is not justifiable, while others believe that *H. pylori* infection should be treated whenever found. The arguments pro and con this view are at

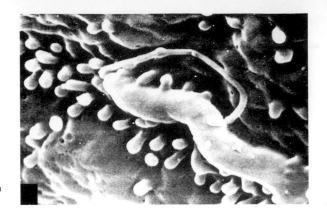

Fig. 1.1 Electron micrograph showing spiral-shaped bacilli in the stomach of a patient with a peptic ulcer.

present theoretical, as there is no evidence for benefit accruing from either course of management. In selected cases of NUD, for example where symptoms are severe, or respond well to acid suppressive agents, *H. pylori* eradication is justifiable on an empirical basis, and may relieve symptoms in the occasional patient.

Gastric cancer is the most serious consequence of *H. pylori* infection

Gastric cancer is the most serious and important consequence of *H. pylori* infection. The bacterium is probably not carcinogenic *per se*, but it sets the scene for cancer to develop. Large scale eradication programmes designed to decrease the incidence of gastric cancer are not feasible at the present stage of *H. pylori* therapy and will probably have to await the availability of a safe, effective and cheap vaccine. There are clinical circumstances when the cancer risk constitutes an indication for treatment, for example in *H. pylori*-positive patients with first-degree relatives with gastric cancer, in those with gastric mucosal risk factors (presence of gastric atrophy, intestinal metaplasia or dysplasia), or in those with fear of cancer who ask for treatment. Patients with mucosa-associated lymphoid tissue lymphoma (MALT), and those with Ménétrier's disease, qualify for treatment.

H. pylori-positive patients on long-term therapy with proton pump inhibitors (PPIs) (e.g. for gastro-oesophageal reflux disease) may have exacerbation of fundic gastritis because of migration of *H. pylori* to that region of the stomach. Eradication could be considered in such cases. There is no unequivocal evidence that NSAID-associated ulcers are related to *H. pylori*. Eradication may be given to patients on NSAIDs with established GU or DU, but this is not a substitute for the treatment of such ulcers on their own merits.

Patient counselling is
essential for good
compliance

All patients given eradication treatment need careful counselling to ensure good compliance, which is fundamental to the
success of therapy. Side effects and future management in event
of treatment failure need to be discussed.

Medical literature is cluttered with a very large number of
treatment trials. Most of these trials comprise small numbers
of patients, many are uncontrolled, very few are blinded, some
are not randomised and most appear only as abstracts and
suffer from multiple publication and piecemeal analysis. To
compound the confusion, numerous regimens that vary in
choice of agents, dose and formulation have been studied. It is
only recently that large, controlled, randomised trials are
beginning to appear. There are very few head-to-head com-
parisons of different treatments.

It therefore is not possible to issue firm guidelines as to
which therapy is the most preferable. Indeed, it is possible that
the results of several available regimens are very similar and

Cost, side effects and
prevalence of
metronidazole-resistant
strains influence the
choice of regimen

the choice will depend on other factors, such as cost, incidence
of side effects, or the prevalence of metronidazole-resistant
strains in the community. The two most important factors that
determine the efficacy of a given treatment regimen are compliance and the prevalence of metronidazole-resistant strains.

Treatment regimens are conveniently classified according to
the number of therapeutic agents. Monotherapy should never
be used because of low efficacy and rapid emergence of bacterial resistance.

Most dual or triple therapy regimens incorporate an acid
suppressive agent, which is either a PPI or a histamine H_2
receptor antagonist (H_2RA). The exception is the 'classical'
bismuth-based triple therapy, comprising bismuth, metronidazole and either ampicillin or tetracycline.

Dual therapy with a PPI and either amoxycillin or clarithromycin eradicates 60–80% of H. pylori, but the results
tend to be variable and highly dependent on compliance. A
variant of dual therapy is a combination of ranitidine and
bismuth which is administered with an antibiotic, usually
clarithromycin. Early data with 2 weeks' treatment look
promising.

Classical bismuth-based triple therapy does not involve acid
suppression. However, the patient is asked to take 11 tablets
daily for 2 weeks, with appreciable incidence of side effects
and a 50% success rate against metronidazole-resistant H.
pylori.

Low-dose, 1-week, triple
therapy regimens are
highly effective

Low-dose triple therapy comprising an acid suppressing agent and two antimicrobials, administered for 1 week, appears to be the best choice at present. The original regimen comprised a PPI, clarithromycin and tinidazole (metronidazole can be used), but larger trials with slightly different dose regimens have now been published and the results will be discussed in some detail. One-week, low-dose triple therapy cures 85–95% of infected patients and is of proven efficacy in metronidazole-resistant strains. A PPI is used in most regimens, but there are some indications that a H_2RA may also be effective.

Quadruple regimens are best reserved for treatment failure due to metronidazole-resistant strains.

Low-dose triple therapy provides a safe and effective treatment for *H. pylori* colonisation of the foregut. It is difficult to see how the present results can be improved with the existing antimicrobial agents. Further advances will probably come from new therapeutic modalities, directed against the toxins expressed by *H. pylori*, or from an effective, cheap and safe vaccine.

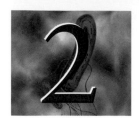

Epidemiology

Summary

- *H. pylori* is probably the most common human chronic infection.
- Humans are the only host for *H. pylori*, which is distributed world-wide.
- Prevalence of *H. pylori* is much higher in emergent countries, or in immigrants from these areas than in the West, where the percentage prevalence of *H. pylori* approximately equals the decade of life.
- The infection is acquired in childhood and persists for life.
- The mode of transmission from person to person is not known. Oral–faecal, oral–oral and gastro-oral routes have all been considered, but not proven.
- The strongest risk factor for acquisition of *H. pylori* infection is socioeconomic deprivation.

Introduction

An understanding of the epidemiology of *H. pylori* infection is necessary to allow us to develop public health measures that will control the spread of the bacterium. A large number of predominantly cross-sectional studies have provided information about the prevalence and risk factors associated with *H. pylori* infection. *H. pylori* infection has a world-wide prevalence, but surprisingly, the route of transmission is still uncertain.

H. pylori has a world-wide prevalence but the route of transmission is uncertain

Host

Humans are the only host for *H. pylori*, where it is found beneath the mucus layer of the gastric epithelium in the stomach. The bacterium is also found on areas of metaplastic gastric epithelium, which may be present in the duodenal bulb, oesophagus, Meckel's diverticulum and rectum, the duodenal bulb location being by far the most important clinically. *H. pylori* has been isolated occasionally in different animal species, including the rhesus monkey, pig, baboon and domestic cat. However, there is no evidence that individuals with domestic cats, or those in contact with other animals, are more likely to be colonised by *H. pylori*; thus, a zoonotic reservoir for *H. pylori* seems unlikely.

Other *Helicobacter* species have been cultured successfully from animals. *H. mustelae* has been found in ferrets, *H. felis* in cats and *H. acinonyx* in cheetahs. There are a number of shared characteristics between the *H. mustelae*-infected ferret and the *H. pylori*-infected human, which have allowed the development of an animal model to study *Helicobacter* infection. In particular, ferrets develop gastritis in response to *H. mustelae* infection and, in some cases, ulceration has been described at the pyloro-duodenal junction. *H. mustelae* adheres firmly to the gastric epithelium in a similar way to *H. pylori*. A mouse model using *H. felis* has also been widely used in the development of a vaccine (see Chapter 7).

Prevalence

The prevalence of *H. pylori* infection increases with age in all population cohorts studied, the prevalence being higher by about 1% per year of age in developed countries. *H. pylori* infection has a world-wide distribution, but is much more common in developing countries. In developed countries *H. pylori* infection is relatively rare in children, with a gradual rise in prevalence with increasing age, reaching 70% in the seventh decade (Fig. 2.1). By contrast, in developing countries childhood infection is commonly present in children and more than 50% of the population are infected by the age of 10 years.

The progressive rise in seroprevalence of *H. pylori* with age could indicate that infection becomes more common as people get older and continue at risk of being colonised by the organism. An alternative theory is that the infection is acquired in childhood. Living circumstances in the past led to more individuals than now becoming infected early in life — the birth–cohort effect. This idea is supported by the observation that acquisition of *H. pylori* during adult life is rare — at least in the West. If this hypothesis is true, then in developed countries the high prevalence of *H. pylori* infection in the older population reflects adverse socioeconomic conditions prevailing at

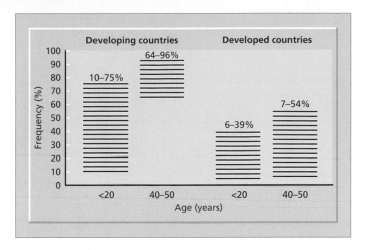

Fig. 2.1 The prevalence of *H. pylori* infection in two age groups (<20 years versus 40–50 years) in developed and developing countries. Factors influencing prevalence: age and socioeconomic status. (Reproduced with permission from Rathbone BJ, Heatley RV. *Helicobacter pylori and Gastroduodenal Disease*. Oxford: Blackwell Science, 1992.)

the beginning of the 20th century; the low prevalence in children at present reflects the current high socioeconomic status. Elderly individuals alive now in developed countries may have been exposed in their childhood to conditions somewhat resembling those that now exist in developing countries. Studies on adults in the Netherlands show an annual *H. pylori*-positive seroconversion rate of less than 0.5%. In developing countries, *H. pylori* infection is acquired during early childhood. This translates into high adult *H. pylori* prevalence, so that by the age of 20 years more than 80% of the population are infected.

Once acquired, *H. pylori* infection is chronic, probably persisting for the individual's lifespan, unless accidentally eradicated by antibiotics given for another reason. Sometimes gastric atrophy, which is the result of colonisation of the gastric mucosa by some strains of *Helicobacter*, progresses to such an extent that the organism is deprived of its habitat and disappears from the stomach. The chronicity of the *H. pylori* infection is remarkable, considering that the bacterium evokes well-marked humoral and tissue immune responses in the human host which, however, are apparently insufficient to clear it from the foregut.

Childhood infection is common in the developing world

Gastric atrophy due to *H. pylori* infection can eliminate the organism

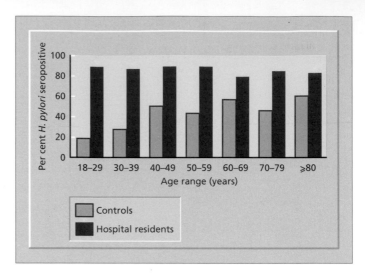

Fig. 2.2 Seroprevalence of *H. pylori* in hospital residents with severe learning difficulties compared with control population. (Reproduced with permission from Harris AW, Douds AC, Meurisse EV *et al*. Seroprevalence of *Helicobacter pylori* in residents of a hospital for people with severe learning difficulties. *Eur J Gastroenterol Hepatol* 1995; **7**: 21–3.)

Risk factors

Low socioeconomic status is linked with an increased risk of infection

The most important risk factor for *H. pylori* besides age is socioeconomic deprivation. Many factors have been researched in this regard, but they all have low economic status as a common denominator. Thus, overcrowding, poor housing, contaminated water supply, bed sharing and large sibships are all implicated. Residence in closed communities, such as homes for the mentally handicapped, long-stay hospitals for the chronically ill or in orphanages, is also a factor; in these circumstances contact between individuals is closer than normal and standards of hygiene may be lower (Fig. 2.2). Thus, *H. pylori* shares attributes with other infections, such as hepatitis A. In fact, it has been remarked that *H. pylori* infection is a better indicator of deprivation than deprivation itself.

Mode of transmission

The mode of transmission of *H. pylori* is unknown. In parallel with other pathogenic bacteria from the gastrointestinal tract, *H. pylori* could be either a strictly human pathogen like

H. pylori transmission
through an environmental
or animal reservoir is
unlikely

Salmonella typhi, acquired from a contaminated environment
or a zoonotic pathogen for which animal reservoirs can be
found. Viable *H. pylori* have never been isolated from the
environment. Investigators from Peru reported finding *H.
pylori* by the polymerase chain reaction (PCR) in sewage
water samples, but these observations have not been confirmed by others. No animal reservoirs for *H. pylori* infection
were thought to exist until recently, when *H. pylori* was
successfully isolated from one group of pathogen-free domestic cats. The presence of *H. pylori* in the gastric mucosa of
these cats was associated with lymphofollicular gastritis,
particularly in the gastric antrum. Moreover, experimental
inoculation of the feline *H. pylori* strain into native cats
without gastric infection led to gastritis identical to that noted
in the naturally infected cats. It is possible that the cats were
infected by transmission from humans, as earlier studies did
not find that cat or pet ownership was a risk factor for *H.
pylori* infection. The significance of this finding is unclear and
unconfirmed at the time of writing. Hence, it seems unlikely
that *H. pylori* is acquired from the environment or from
animals, and person-to-person transmission is more likely. The
latter may occur through oral–oral, gastro-oral or faecal–oral
routes.

Person-to-person
transmission may involve
oral–oral, gastro-oral or
faecal–oral routes

Oral–oral transmission

H. pylori may be transported in gastric juice to the oesophagus
and mouth during regurgitation of gastric contents. Indeed, *H.
pylori* has been found in the gullet in cases of Barrett's oesophagus. However, attempts to culture the bacterium from the
mouth have been mostly unsuccessful, possibly because of
technical difficulties, or because the bacterium is only a tem-
porary resident in the buccal cavity. *H. pylori* DNA has been
detected using PCR and other techniques in human saliva and
dental plaque. An interesting study using restriction endo-
nuclease analysis of dental and gastric colonies of *H. pylori*
from one patient showed these to be the same clone, raising the
possibility that the mouth may act as a reservoir for *H. pylori*.
In a study from western Africa, where the baby's food is pre-
masticated by the mother, an association between *H. pylori*
infection and pre-mastication was found, supporting a potential role of oral–oral transmission of *H. pylori*. These preliminary findings need confirmation before conclusions regarding
the importance of oral–oral spread can be drawn. At present,

There is some evidence
to support oral–oral
transmission, but its
importance has yet to be
established

there is no epidemiological evidence to suggest that the oral–oral route is important.

Gastro-oral transmission

It has been suggested that *H. pylori* may be transmitted between individuals in vomitus. *H. pylori* has been cultured successfully from gastric juice. Vomiting and regurgitation is common in childhood and it is possible that the bacterium may spread between children (or children and adults) in vomitus.

In two well-documented human *H. pylori* ingestion studies, the volunteers drank a solution containing live *H. pylori* and were closely monitored thereafter. In both cases, vomiting occurred after colonisation of the stomach by *H. pylori*. These studies lend credence to the interesting hypothesis that *H. pylori* may be transmitted through a gastro-oral route, which could explain the acquisition of *H. pylori* early in life. The reported transmission of *H. pylori* by contaminated endoscopes or nasogastric tubes after inadequate sterilisation may involve a similar mechanism. Seroepidemiological data also highlight the risk of gastro-oral contamination. The prevalence of *H. pylori* infection in gastroenterologists, determined by an immunoglobulin G (IgG) enzyme-linked immunosorbent assay (ELISA), was significantly higher than the prevalence found in age-matched blood donors, general practitioners and endoscopy nurses. The discrepancy with the latter group may be explained by the fact that only 9% of gastroenterologists wore gloves, compared with 72% of the nurses studied.

Vomiting stimulated by H. pylori colonisation may contribute to gastro-oral transmission

Faecal–oral transmission

Culture of *H. pylori* from the faeces of infected dyspeptic patients in the UK and from infected malnourished children in Gambia has been reported. However, other investigators have been unable to confirm these findings. *H. pylori* has been detected in faeces using PCR, but this finding does not discriminate between viable and dead bacteria. Even though *H. pylori* has been detected in faeces, the significance of these findings is unclear at present and viable organisms have not been shown unequivocally to be present in human stools. *H. pylori* infection is not associated with diarrhoea.

The faecal–oral transmission route remains unconfirmed

Epidemiological studies from Thailand and France have indicated that the prevalence of hepatitis A infection parallels that of *H. pylori* infection. Hepatitis A is known to be transmitted via a faecal–oral route, and these findings support the hypothesis that *H. pylori* infection is spread by a similar mechanism.

Re-infection

In developed countries re-infection after successful eradication is very uncommon and probably no more than between 0.5 and 1.5% each year. Re-infection may be higher in children due to the presence of risk factors present in this age group, such as lower standards of hygiene and close physical proximity (sharing bedrooms). As discussed above, socioeconomic conditions are of utmost importance in determining the prevalence of *H. pylori* infection. In developing countries where family sizes are large, standards of hygiene are low and overcrowding is commonplace, the risk of re-infection with *H. pylori* may be higher than that reported from the industrialised nations, and may be as high as 50% each year.

Further epidemiological studies are needed to establish the route of transmission

It is remarkable that despite world-wide distribution and high prevalence, the route of transmission of *H. pylori* remains to be worked out.

Further reading

Axon ATR. The transmission of *Helicobacter pylori*: which theory fits the facts? *Eur J Gastroenterol Hepatol* 1996; 8(1): 1–2.

Mégraud F. Epidemiology of *Helicobacter pylori* infection: where are we in 1995? *Eur J Gastroenterol Hepatol* 1995; 7: 292–5.

Mendall MA, Goggin PM, Molineaux N *et al*. Childhood living conditions and *Helicobacter pylori* seropositivity in adult life. *Lancet* 1992; **332**: 896–7.

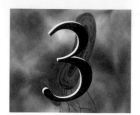

Pathophysiology

Summary

• Bacterial and host factors, which are still imperfectly understood, determine the outcome of *H. pylori* infection. *H. pylori* strains that are *cag*A positive are associated with pathology. *H. pylori* infection evokes immune reaction in the host, but this is insufficient to clear the infection.

• Most *H. pylori*-colonised subjects develop superficial gastritis, which has no clinical consequences.

• In some subjects *H. pylori* infection may mainly affect the antrum and produce antritis.

• *H. pylori* antritis is associated with hypergastrinaemia and high acid output. There is an increased risk of duodenal ulcer and a decreased risk of intestinal-type gastric cancer.

• Hypersecretion of acid leads to gastric metaplasia in the duodenum, which may become colonised by *H. pylori*, with subsequent duodenitis and ulcer formation.

• In others, *H. pylori* may mainly colonise the corpus, producing atrophic gastritis, low acid secretion and an increased risk of gastric ulcer and of intestinal type of gastric cancer.

Re-interpretation of gastric pathophysiology in duodenal ulcer (DU) disease in the *H. pylori* era

Many abnormalities of gastric function have been described in patients with DU. All the data and concepts acquired previously and published in the voluminous literature need to be re-examined and re-interpreted in the light of recent knowledge pertaining to the way in which *H. pylori* infection affects gastric function. Gastric activities affected by the bacterium include secretion of antral polypeptide hormones, gastric acid secretion, the distribution of gastric-type mucosa and its inflammatory response to infection. Interpretation of older data is made difficult, or impossible in numerous instances, because subjects and controls were selected without the

H. pylori infection alters stomach function at the cellular level

Table 3.1 Abnormalities of gastric function associated with DU.

Increased postprandial and bombesin-stimulated plasma gastrin concentrations

Increased parietal cell mass (increased pentagastrin-stimulated maximal or peak acid output)

Peak acid output approximately twice the normal level

Increased basal, meal- and bombesin/gastrin releasing peptide (GRP)-stimulated acid output

Defective inhibitory control of acid secretion: meal-stimulated secretion less inhibited by low intragastric pH, intraduodenal fat or gastric antral distension

Fewer somatostatin-containing antral D cells

Bombesin/GRP are closely related neuropeptides which mediate release of gastrin from antral G cells and somatostatin from antral D cells (see p. 19).

knowledge of their *H. pylori* status. Abnormalities of gastric function reported in patients with DU are listed in Table 3.1.

The result of these recognised abnormalities is excess secretion of acid. Surgery used to be the only potentially curative treatment for patients with chronic DU disease and a wide range of operations, such as partial gastrectomy to remove the antrum (reduces gastrin production) and a variable portion of the corpus (removes parietal cells), or highly selective vagotomy (denervates acid–pepsin secretion) were performed. However, in the 1970s the discovery of histamine H_2 receptor antagonists (H_2RAs) and in the 1980s the discovery of proton pump inhibitors (PPIs), both of which decrease acid output and heal DU, revolutionised the medical treatment of DU disease and re-emphasised the importance of gastric acid in the aetiology of DU. Environmental factors, such as stress, cigarettes, and spicy food ('worry, hurry, curry'), were thought to exacerbate DU disease and increase the likelihood of relapse. However, since the discovery of *H. pylori* and its link with DU disease, investigators have re-evaluated these abnormalities of gastric physiology in patients with DU to determine the aetiological role of *H. pylori*.

H. pylori is present in the gastric antrum in more than 95% of patients who are not using non-steroidal anti-inflammatory drugs (NSAIDs), suggesting that infection with *H. pylori* is an essential prerequisite of DU disease. Furthermore, eradication of *H. pylori* profoundly changes the natural history of DU disease by reducing the incidence of relapse from 80% to less than 2% each year. Detailed knowledge of the mechanisms through which *H. pylori* infection of the stomach

Raised acid secretion has been treated with surgery, H_2-histamine blockers or PPIs

Over 95% of non-NSAID DU patients are colonised with *H. pylori*

13 / Pathophysiology

eventually causes DU in a minority of people colonised by the organism is expanding very rapidly, but is not complete at present. However, there are a number of areas where the pathophysiology of DU has recently become much clearer. There is also good documentation in the literature of reversal of abnormalities and return to normal of various aspects of gastric function after eradication of the bacterium.

Host response

Gastritis

Infection with *H. pylori* is now accepted as the cause of almost all non-immune chronic gastritis. Eradication of *H. pylori* leads to healing of the gastritis and the return of the antral and body mucosa to normal histology. Following colonisation of the foregut by *H. pylori*, mucosal lesions take years to develop and progress: in most subjects chronic superficial gastritis is the only outcome, which has no clinical significance.

The gastritis can be antral-predominant, or corpus-predominant, or can affect both parts of the stomach (pangastritis) (Figs 3.1 & 3.2). The distribution of *H. pylori* within the stomach appears to be very important, because this feature probably determines the clinical manifestation of disease. The factors that determine the distribution of *H. pylori*, and thus of the gastritis, within the stomach are at present unclear.

One hypothesis states that the most important factor in the distribution of *H. pylori* in the stomach is local acid produc-

Colonisation of the foregut with *H. pylori* mainly results in gastritis only

H. pylori distribution in the stomach determines clinical manifestations

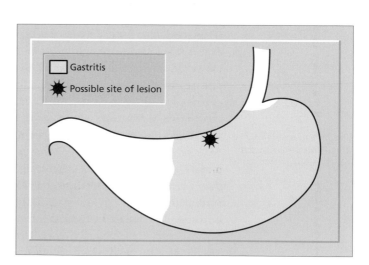

Fig. 3.1 The pattern of gastritis in gastric ulcer (GU): body gastritis.

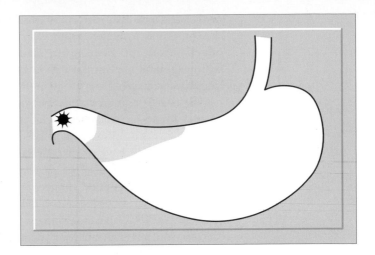

Fig. 3.2 The pattern of gastritis in DU: antral gastritis. Use of colour explained in Fig. 3.1.

The link between level of acid secretion and colonisation pattern may explain the geographical variation in gastro-duodenal disorders

tion. Thus, in individuals with low acid secretion, possibly secondary to poor general nutrition, intercurrent illness and colonisation of the stomach by micro-organisms (conditions likely to prevail in emergent countries), *H. pylori* will colonise the antrum and body of the stomach, inducing inflammation (gastritis) at both sites. This may eventually result in gastric ulcer (GU) and, possibly, gastric corpus mucosal atrophy, with associated increased risk of gastric cancer. In other individuals with a high acid output, possibly genetically determined, or in areas of high standards of hygiene and nutrition (conditions likely to prevail in industrialised countries), *H. pylori* preferentially colonises the antrum, where it may increase acid secretion from parietal cells in the gastric corpus (see p. 21).

This increased acid output may increase the prevalence and extent of gastric metaplasia in the duodenal bulb and thereby allow the bacterium to colonise it, which may in turn lead to DU in some individuals. *H. pylori* will not fluorish in the gastric body under these circumstances and these individuals will remain at low risk for GU and gastric cancer. This hypothesis goes some way towards explaining the different patterns of gastritis recognised in patients with DU or GU (Figs 3.1 & 3.2) and the spectrum of *H. pylori*-associated gastroduodenal diseases found in different populations. The gastritis associated with DU predominantly affects the antrum, although mild or moderate inflammation of the corpus can be present. Glandular atrophy in the gastric body or fundus is absent or mild, and intestinal metaplasia is rare. Pre-pyloric GU is also associated with this pattern of gastritis. By contrast, chronic benign GU is associated with gastritis involving corpus and antral mucosa in a pangastritis. Glandular atrophy and intestinal metaplasia are common findings; their degree and extent increases with age.

The antral-predominant gastritis with relative sparing of the corpus found in patients with DU or pre-pyloric GU means that the parietal cell mass is unaffected by atrophy and these patients tend to have normal or high gastric acid secretion. This is not only because the parietal cell mass is spared, but also because of profound changes induced by *H. pylori* in the endocrine function of the antral mucosa. On the other hand, patients with GU have multifocal atrophy of antrum and corpus, which is associated with decreased acid secretion and a low risk of DU, and, if gastric atrophy supervenes, with an increased risk of distal gastric cancer.

Gastric metaplasia and duodenitis

Gastric metaplasia — the replacement of the columnar cells which normally cover the duodenal villi by gastric-type epithelium rich in neutral mucin — is present in more than 90% of patients with DU, but in only about 50% of healthy subjects. *H. pylori* is able to colonise only gastric-type epithelium with its overlying layer of mucus, and the presence of gastric metaplasia makes it possible for *H. pylori* to colonise the duodenal bulb (Plate 3.1, facing p. 26). Colonisation of the duodenal bulb by *H. pylori* leads to mucosal inflammation (duodenitis), which makes the gastric mucosal islands in the duodenal bulb vulnerable to attack by acid and/or pepsin, or bile, with subsequent ulceration. Exactly how *H. pylori* travels from the antral to the gastric metaplastic mucosa in the duodenal bulb is not clear. Motility of the organism, which can be demonstrated clearly and measured under experimental conditions, may be very important here.

The factors that determine the presence and extent of gastric metaplasia in the duodenal bulb are unclear. Gastric metaplasia may be a protective response of the duodenal epithelium to injury. Animal models indicate that gastric metaplasia develops in the presence of duodenal injury and gastric acid. Human studies are less clear-cut. It has been shown that the prevalence and extent of duodenal gastric metaplasia correlates positively with gastric acid output, which may explain why gastric metaplasia is so much more common and greater in extent in

Gastric metaplasia enables *H. pylori* to colonise the duodenal bulb

High acid output stimulates the development of gastric metaplasia patients with DU, than in healthy subjects. The secretion of mucus by the columnar epithelium may delay the diffusion of hydrogen ions (H^+), allowing time for secreted mucosal bicarbonate to neutralise acid, and thereby protect the underlying epithelium from low pH and damage.

H. *pylori* may increase the prevalence and extent of gastric metaplasia in the duodenal bulb by increasing the amount of acid arriving in the duodenal bulb (see p. 24), and by inducing an inflammatory response in the duodenal mucosa adjacent to islands of metaplasia through the release of inflammatory mediators.

Bacterial factors

Adhesion

H. pylori colonises gastric-type epithelium only, by resting under mucus on the cell surface

H. *pylori* can colonise only gastric-type epithelium and is not found in the normal duodenum, nor anywhere else in the gastrointestinal tract in the absence of gastric mucosa. The organism is superbly adapted to its ecological niche, resting on the surface of gastric epithelial cells beneath the layer of mucus. The spiral shape and motility conferred by its multiple flagella may help to distribute it over the gastric mucosa. H. *pylori* adhere to the epithelial cell surface, a process which may involve pedestal formation. This adherence is characteristic of pathogenic bacteria. For example, one of the major characteristics differentiating enteropathic from non-enteropathic *Escherichia coli* is the ability of the former to adhere to an epithelial surface.

Toxins

Type I H. pylori *release the toxin VacA*

H. *pylori*, like other pathogenic bacteria, causes tissue damage by releasing toxins. H. *pylori* strains can be divided phenotypically into two groups. One group (type I) contains the 94-kDa VacA- (the vacuolating toxin, encoded by the gene *vac*A) and the 120–128-kDa CagA- (cytotoxin-associated protein, encoded by the gene *cag*A) expressing strains; the second group (type II) contains non-cytotoxic, VacA-negative and CagA-negative strains. There is evidence that type I strains trigger more intensive inflammation than type II.

About 60% of strains of H. *pylori* produce a vacuolating toxin, which vacuolates cultured cells *in vitro*. Interestingly, the production of vacuolating toxin may be related to the clini-

There is a high correlation
between DU and strains
that produce vacuolating
toxin

cal manifestation of *H. pylori* infection. It has been reported that about 70% of strains from patients with DU produce this toxin, compared with only about 30% of strains from patients with non-ulcer dyspepsia. Antibodies to CagA and to VacA (type I) are also more common among patients with DU than in non-ulcer patients. Infection with strains expressing VacA and CagA is associated with the increased secretion of inter-leukin-8 (IL-8) by gastric epithelial cells, which may have a key role in *H. pylori*-induced mucosal inflammation. In addition to attracting neutrophils, IL-8 may stimulate gastrin release from antral G cells. Thus, *H. pylori*-induced release of IL-8 may contribute to the increased gastrin release recorded in patients infected with *H. pylori*. There is some evidence to suggest that the degree of inflammation, and possibly the clinical conse-quence of *H. pylori* infection, are related to the density of bac-terial colonisation of the stomach.

Degree of inflammation
may be related to density
of colonisation

Table 3.2 Clinical consequences of infection with different strains of *H. pylori*.

H. pylori strain	VacA positive	VacA negative
	CagA positive	CagA negative
Genotype	vacA (type s1) positive	vacA positive
	cagA positive	cagA negative
Toxin	Vacuolating toxin	None
Disease association	DU more likely	DU less likely

Specific *H. pylori* *vac*A genotypes that are associated with peptic ulceration and the degree of inflammation have been described recently (Table 3.2). *vac*A, the gene encoding the vacuolating cytotoxin, has a mosaic structure consisting of one of three signal sequence types (s1a, s1b and s2), and one of two mid-region types (m1 and m2). Type s1 strains were signifi-cantly more common than type s2 strains in patients with a past or present history of DU. Furthermore, type s1a strains were associated with greater neutrophil density than type s1b or s2 strains. *vac*A mid-region typing did not appear to be associated with DU disease, inflammation or bacterial density. Thus, specific *vac*A signal sequence types may be associated with the ability of *H. pylori* strains to cause peptic ulceration.

Urease

H. pylori abundantly expresses a nickel-containing urease enzyme, which hydrolyses urea into ammonia with net pro-duction of alkali. This process thus may produce a neutral microenvironment for the organism. Urease may have a role in *H. pylori* metabolism as part of the nitrogen cycle. It has been suggested that the ammonia generated by the *H. pylori* urease may work with the cytotoxin in inducing vacuoles, because it has been shown that urease-negative mutant strains of *H. pylori* do not produce them.

Inflammation

H. pylori is strongly antigenic, leading to humoral (IgG and IgA) and cellular immune responses. Despite mounting a vigorous immune response the human host is unable to clear *H. pylori*, which persists for a very long time, perhaps for the lifetime of the infected individual. *H. pylori* induces an inflammatory response in the gastric mucosa by producing substances which attract and activate neutrophils. The inflammatory response leads to the accumulation of a number of different cytokines, including IL-8 and tumour necrosis factor α (TNF-α). In patients with DU these two cytokines play an important role in the formation of the inflammatory infiltrate affecting mainly the gastric antrum, which resolves completely after eradication of *H. pylori*.

The inflammatory
response to *H. pylori*
involves IL-8 and TNF-α

   H.-pylori strains may vary in their ability to stimulate the gastric epithelium to express IL-8. Thus, type I *H. pylori* (VacA positive, CagA positive) and type s1a *vac*A strains have been shown to induce significantly higher IL-8 levels than type II and type s1b or s2 strains. In the future it may be possible as part of routine clinical practice to identify the particular strain that colonises an individual and thus determine the likelihood of developing DU disease, or even gastric cancer.

Effect of *H. pylori* on gastric secretory function

Gastrin

Gastrin is a peptide hormone produced by G cells found mainly in the antrum of the stomach. Gastrin stimulates parietal cells to secrete acid. The stimulation of acid secretion by gastrin is probably induced indirectly by enhancement of histamine release from enterochromaffin-like (ECL) cells in the fundic mucosa, rather than by a direct effect on gastrin receptors on the parietal cell (Fig. 3.3). In addition to stimulating acid secretion, gastrin has a trophic action on mucosal cells, including parietal cells. A negative feedback mechanism stimu-

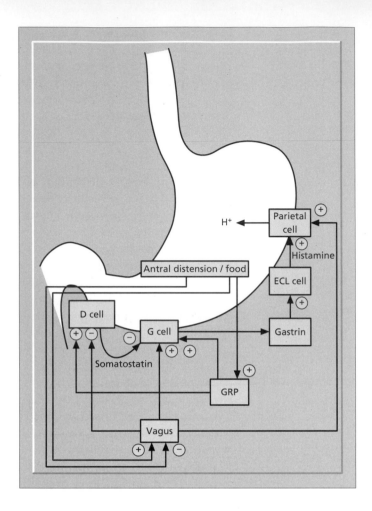

Fig. 3.3 The relationship between D, G and parietal cells in the stomach.

lates gastrin release from the antral G cells whenever antral pH rises; gastrin release is inhibited by the presence of antral acidification (pH < 3) (Fig. 3.3). Control of gastrin release is additionally mediated through local paracrine effect of somatostatin, a polypeptide inhibitory hormone produced by the so-called D cells in the gastric antrum. There may also be some direct effect of H^+ on the antral G cells, or interference by acid with the mucosal uptake of amino acids necessary for gastrin release.

> Gastrin release is controlled by somatostatin and modulated by acid

H. pylori infection is associated with increased fasting serum gastrin concentrations in healthy subjects and in patients with DU. When compared with *H. pylori*-negative healthy subjects, *H. pylori*-positive individuals have increased basal, meal- and GRP-stimulated serum gastrin (GRP is a 27 amino acid peptide

> *H. pylori* infection is associated with increased serum gastrin levels

which mediates release of gastrin from antral G cells, and also stimulates the release of gastric inhibitory peptides such as somatostatin and cholecystokinin). *H. pylori* eradication is followed within 2 weeks by complete resolution of the hypergastrinaemia, which is mostly due to a selective increase in gastrin-17 (consisting of 17 amino acid residues), the predominant form of gastrin in the antrum.

Somatostatin

Antral somatostatin concentration and D-cell density are lower in the antral mucosa of *H. pylori*-positive than in *H. pylori*-negative patients

Somatostatin secreted from the antral D cells is the main inhibitor of exocrine and endocrine secretion by the stomach and exerts a tonic restraint on acid secretion through actions on antral G cells, parietal cells and fundal histamine-containing cells (Fig. 3.3).

The important observation in the present context is that antral somatostatin concentrations and D-cell density are significantly lower in the antral mucosa of *H. pylori*-positive patients with DU than in *H. pylori*-negative subjects. After eradication of *H. pylori*, antral somatostatin content and D-cell density return to the normal range. This suggests that the

Hypergastrinaemia in *H. pylori*-positive DU is due to somatostatin deficiency

hypergastrinaemia found in *H. pylori*-positive patients with DU is due to a deficiency of antral D-cell somatostatin, which normally tonically inhibits the synthesis and release of gastrin (Fig. 3.3). Thus, somatostatin seems to be a key hormone modulating (through gastrin) gastric acid secretion and (through the trophic effect of gastrin) the size of the parietal cell mass in patients with DU. Inflammatory changes induced by *H. pylori* profoundly affect the metabolism of somatostatin and hence secretory aspects of gastric function.

Histamine

Mucosal levels of histamine are reduced with *H. pylori* infection

H. pylori infection in patients with DU is associated with decreased gastric body mucosal histamine, either because of enhanced histamine release or low synthesis by ECL and mast cells. *H. pylori* has been shown to induce histamine release from human mast cells by an IgE-mediated reaction and, in addition, the inflammatory response to *H. pylori* itself may release histamine from mast cells. It has been reported recently that *H. pylori* possesses an enzyme which produces a potent agonist at histamine H_3 receptors ($N\alpha$-methyl histamine). These receptors are involved in the regulation of acid and somatostatin secretion, and exert negative feedback on hista-

21 / Pathophysiology

mine synthesis and release. Thus, production of this agonist by *H. pylori* may lead to decreased histamine synthesis (which might account for the low antral histamine content found in *H. pylori*-positive patients with DU) and an inhibitory effect on the somatostatin content of antral D cells.

In summary, *H. pylori* changes the regulation of acid secretion in two opposite ways: its effect on fundic histamine formation can decrease acid secretion, but the effect on antral somatostatin induces hypergastrinaemia and increases gastric acid output. The final result on acid secretion depends on the balance of these factors; they in turn are governed by the extent and distribution of *H. pylori* infection in the stomach (see p. 14). These important observations go a long way towards explaining the hyperacidity associated with DU, as in this disease *H. pylori* predominantly colonises the antrum, with consequent antritis. Corpusitis, accompanied by hypoacidity, is the predominant lesion in GU or cancer. It is remarkable that, as far as it is known at present, all the abnormalities of gastric function revert to normality after successful treatment of *H. pylori* infection. This observation has profound clinical importance and explains not only the healing of DU or GU after *H. pylori* eradication, but also the highly significantly decreased risk of relapse of peptic ulcer. It may also provide a basis for the prevention of those types of gastric cancer that are associated with *H. pylori* infection.

Effect of *H. pylori* on gastric acid output

Gastric acid secretion is measured using basal and stimulated outputs

The importance of the changes in somatostatin, gastrin and histamine metabolism discussed above, depends on the subsequent changes in gastric acid secretion. The most commonly used measurements of gastric acid secretion are basal and stimulated acid outputs. Basal acid output is the amount of acid secreted under resting, unstimulated conditions. Maximal or peak acid output is best determined after stimulation with pentagastrin, a synthetic pentapeptide analogue of gastrin. Pentagastrin stimulates acid secretion by the parietal cells, probably through the release of histamine from ECL or mast cells in the fundic mucosa. Thus, pentagastrin-stimulated peak acid output is a measure of the total functional parietal cell mass of the stomach. Another stimulant of gastric acid secretion is the neuropeptide, GRP. GRP stimulates the release of gastrin from antral G cells, but at the same time it stimulates the release of inhibitory peptides, such as somatostatin, from antral D cells.

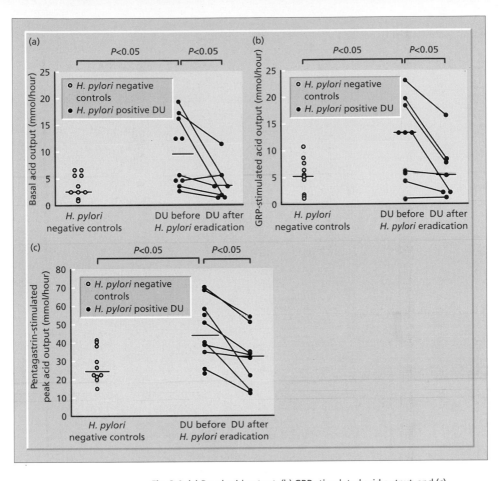

Fig. 3.4 (a) Basal acid output, (b) GRP-stimulated acid output, and (c) pentagastrin-stimulated peak acid output in controls and patients with DU before and after eradication of *H. pylori*. (Reproduced with permission from Harris AW, Gummett PA, Misiewicz JJ, Baron JH. Eradication of *Helicobacter pylori* in patients with duodenal ulcer lowers basal and peak acid outputs to gastrin releasing peptide and pentagastrin. *Gut* 1996; **38**: 663–7.)

GRP-stimulated acid output is thus a measure of the combined functional response of the body (parietal cells) to endogenous gastrin released by antral G cells, after modulation by somatostatin (from antral D cells) (Fig. 3.3). This stimulation using GRP may mimic the effect that eating a meal has on gastric secretory function.

Basal, GRP- and pentagastrin-stimulated peak acid outputs are significantly higher in *H. pylori*-positive patients with DU than in *H. pylori*-negative healthy controls (Fig. 3.4). Basal and pentagastrin-stimulated peak acid outputs in *H. pylori*-

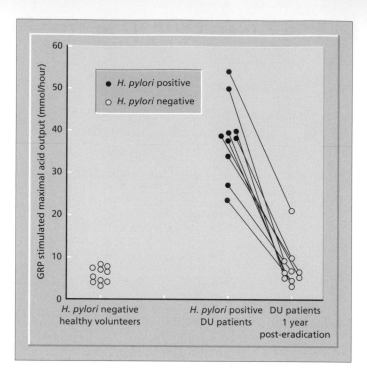

Fig. 3.5 Calculated maximal acid output to GRP stimulation in the various groups of subjects studied. Values in *H. pylori*-positive patients with DUs are higher than those in the *H. pylori*-negative volunteers (*P* < 0.001), but decrease to a similar level to the volunteers 1 year after eradication. (Reproduced with permission from El-Omar E, Penman ID, Ardill JES *et al. Helicobacter pylori* and abnormalities of acid secretion in patients with duodenal ulcer disease. *Gastroenterology* 1995; **109**(3): 681–91.)

High acid output is reduced significantly after *H. pylori* eradication therapy

positive patients with DU are about twice that of normal, while GRP-stimulated acid output is increased between three- and sixfold. All these measurements of acid output have been shown to decrease significantly after eradication of *H. pylori* in patients with DU (Fig. 3.4). The decreased basal and pentagastrin-stimulated peak acid output reflect decreases in the parietal cell mass after eradication of *H. pylori* and the removal of trophic drive due to hypergastrinaemia. GRP-stimulated acid output was shown to decrease by 66% 1 month after eradication of *H. pylori*, and to return to normal by the end of 1 year after *H. pylori* eradication (Fig. 3.5). These changes probably result from the return of antral somatostatin levels to normal, with an increase in the inhibitory control of acid secretion.

The changes in basal and stimulated acid output after eradication of *H. pylori* support the hypothesis that *H. pylori* infection impairs the inhibitory control of gastric acid secretion, which is mediated largely through somatostatin. The increased gastric acid secretion may result in increased duodenal acid load and, in the presence of duodenitis secondary to colonisation by *H. pylori*, to ulceration.

Further reading

Crabtree JE, Taylor JD, Wyatt JI *et al*. Mucosal recognition of *Helicobacter pylori* 120 kDa protein, peptic ulceration and gastric pathology. *Lancet* 1991; **338**: 332–5.

Crabtree JE, Wyatt JI, Trejdosiewicz LK *et al*. Interleukin-8 expression in *Helicobacter pylori* infected, normal and neoplastic gastroduodenal mucosa. *J Clin Pathol* 1994; **47**: 61–6.

El-Omar E, Penman I, Dorrian CA *et al*. Eradicating *Helicobacter pylori* infection lowers gastrin-mediated acid secretion by two-thirds in patients with duodenal ulcer. *Gut* 1993; **34**: 1060–5.

Harris AW, Gummett PA, Misiewicz JJ, Baron JH. Eradication of *Helicobacter pylori* in patients with duodenal ulcer lowers basal and peak acid outputs to gastrin releasing peptide and pentagastrin. *Gut* 1996; **38**: 663–7.

Moss SF, Calam J. Acid secretion and sensitivity to gastrin in patients with duodenal ulcer: effect of eradication of *Helicobacter pylori*. *Gut* 1993; **34**: 888–92.

Moss SF, Legon S, Bishop AE *et al*. Effect of *Helicobacter pylori* on gastric somatostatin in duodenal ulcer disease. *Lancet* 1992; **340**: 930–2.

Noach LA, Rolf TM, Bosma NB *et al*. Gastric metaplasia and *Helicobacter pylori* infection. *Gut* 1993; **34**: 1510–14.

Pounder RE. *Helicobacter pylori* and gastroduodenal secretory function. *Gastroenterology* 1996; **110**(3): 947–9.

Wyatt JI, Rathbone BJ, Dixon MF *et al*. *Campylobacter pyloridis* and acid induced gastric metaplasia in the pathogenesis of duodenitis. *J Clin Pathol* 1987; **40**: 841–8.

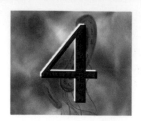

Diagnosis

Summary

• Invasive tests for the diagnosis of *H. pylori* utilise endoscopic biopsies, taken for the urease test, histology or culture.
• The urease test on biopsies provides a rapid and accurate diagnosis of *H. pylori* infection.
• Histology is a reliable, but slower and more expensive diagnostic technique.
• Culture is the gold standard, but fails in a proportion of cases. It is best reserved for problems, for example determination of *H. pylori* resistance to antibiotics.
• Non-invasive tests comprise serology and ^{13}C or ^{14}C-urea breath tests.
• Serology is excellent for screening, but not good for determining the outcome of treatment.
• Breath tests are best for monitoring the result of eradication therapy.

H. pylori infection may be diagnosed by invasive tests at endoscopy or non-invasive tests without endoscopy

As in any other condition, accurate diagnosis is essential before treatment is started, and several techniques are available. *H. pylori* infection may be diagnosed by invasive tests, those requiring upper gastrointestinal endoscopy or by non-invasive tests in which endoscopy is not necessary. Most methods used in the diagnosis have high specificity and sensitivity, but at present there is no agreed gold standard for diagnosing *H. pylori* infection (Table 4.1). It has been suggested that a combination of three separate diagnostic tests is needed to confirm the presence or absence of *H. pylori* infection, but this is not always practical, or indeed necessary. A summary of the individual investigative tests is given in Table 4.1.

Invasive tests

Invasive methods of investigation use gastric biopsies taken

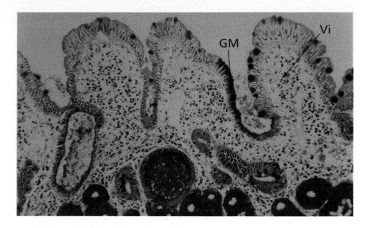

Plate 3.1 Duodenal bulb mucosa showing areas of gastric metaplasia. GM, gastric metaplasia; Vi, villus. PAS, ×55.

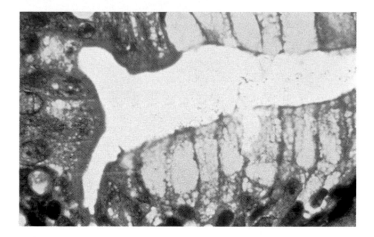

Plate 4.1 Histological appearance of *Helicobacter*-like organisms in a gastric body biopsy, stained with modified Giemsa stain. ×100.

[*Facing on p. 26*]

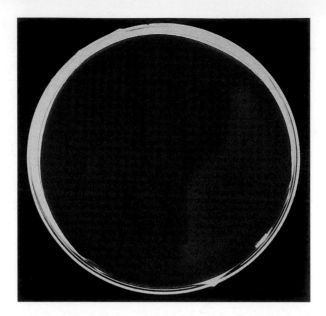

Plate 4.2 Microbiological cultures are used to determine the sensitivity of the bacterium to antibiotics. A metronidazole-impregnated epsilometer (E) strip is placed on an agar plate inoculated with *H. pylori*. The lowest metronidazole concentration that inhibits *H. pylori* is read off the scale (0.25 mg l^{-1}). GIZ, *H. pylori* growth inhibition zone. (Reproduced courtesy of Dr Karim, St Mary's Hospital, London.)

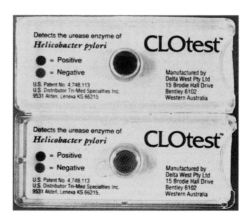

Plate 4.3 *H. pylori*-positive (above) and *H. pylori*-negative CLO™ test.

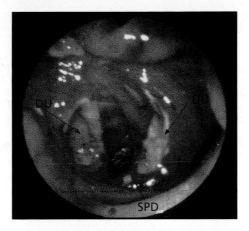

Plate 6.1 Endoscopic appearance of duodenal ulcer (DU). SPD, opening into the second part of the duodenum.

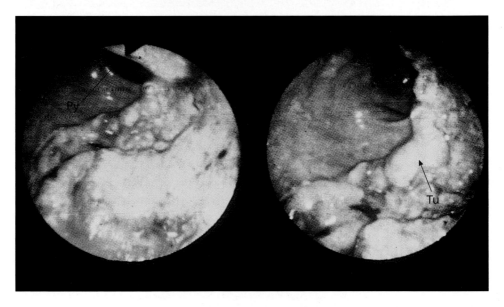

Plate 6.2 Endoscopic appearance of gastric cancer. Py, pylorus; Tu, tumour in antrum.

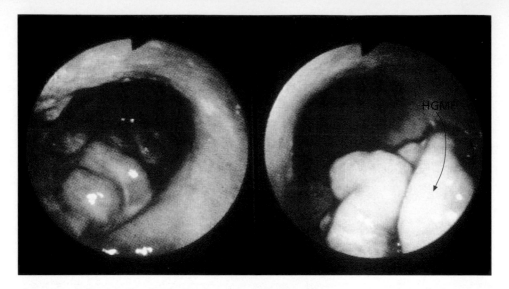

Plate 6.3 Endoscopic appearance of Ménétrier's disease (hypertrophic gastropathy). HGMF, hypertrophic gastric mucosal folds.

Table 4.1 Summary of investigative methods for *H. pylori* diagnosis.

Diagnostic method	Main indication	Sensitivity (%)	Specificity (%)
Histology	Diagnosis	90	95
Culture	*H. pylori* antibiotic sensitivities	80–90	95
Rapid urease test	Endoscopy room diagnosis	90	100
Serology (laboratory based)	Screening and diagnosis	80–90	90
Urea breath test	To confirm eradication	95	100

at endoscopy for histology, bacterial culture, the rapid urease test (CLO™test — CLO stands for 'Campylobacter-like organisms,' an old name for Helicobacter) or the polymerase chain reaction (PCR).

Histology

Endoscopic antral and/or gastric body biopsies are fixed in 10% formalin, routinely processed and stained with haematoxylin and eosin, and a stain of choice to show *Helicobacter*-like organisms (HLOs). This may be a modified Giemsa stain or Gimenez (Plate 4.1, facing p. 26). This method has been shown to be sensitive ($>90\%$) and specific ($>95\%$) for identification of *H. pylori*, but is dependent on the availability of an experienced histopathologist. It is a routine procedure for the endoscopist to obtain mucosal biopsies during the procedure. Histology also provides information concerning the severity of the gastritis and the possible presence of pre-malignant changes, such as intestinal metaplasia or dysplasia of the gastric mucosa. In addition, the absence of chronic antral inflammation (increased numbers of mononuclear cells in the lamina propria) is a highly specific (negative predictive value of 100%) method to exclude *H. pylori* infection.

Histology is highly sensitive and specific, but needs an experienced histopathologist

Bacterial culture

Gastric biopsies are placed in chilled Stuart's transport medium, *Brucella* broth or sterile saline and, within 24 hours, selective and non-selective media, such as brain heart infusion agar with 5% horse defibrinated blood, are inoculated. The plates are incubated using microaerobic (5% oxygen) and hypercapnic (5–10% carbon dioxide (CO_2)) conditions at 37°C for up to 10 days. Identity of *H. pylori* is confirmed by Gram stain and production of urease, oxidase and catalase.

The sensitivity and specificity of this test are greater than 95% and 80–90%, respectively. *H. pylori* is not easy to culture and this method is time consuming and expensive. Even in dedicated laboratories there is an appreciable (20%) incidence of failure of the organism to grow; possibly because of its reduced viability after patients' ingestion of topical anaesthetic, prior treatment with antibiotics, proton pump inhibitors or specimen transport in room air. Although isolation of *H. pylori* in culture certainly indicates its presence, a negative culture does not prove its absence.

H. pylori is a difficult organism to culture

Microbiological culture is indicated when it is necessary to determine the sensitivity of the bacterium to antibiotics; for example, after a failed course of eradication therapy (Plate 4.2, facing p. 26).

Rapid urease test

These tests are dependent on the potent urease enzyme produced by active *H. pylori*, which hydrolyses urea into ammonia (Fig. 4.1). A single gastric biopsy is placed into the well of a CLO™ test slide, but there is some evidence to suggest that the early sensitivity of CLO™ test results can be improved by placing two or more gastric biopsies in the test well. A positive result is indicated by a change in the pH indicator dye colour from yellow to pink (Plate 4.3, facing p. 26). About 80% of *H. pylori*-infected specimens react positively to the CLO™ test within 20 minutes. Specimens with low urease activity may take up to 24 hours to change colour. False-positive result may occasionally occur from other urease-producing organisms (streptococcal and staphylococcal

A colour change from yellow to pink indicates a positive CLO™ test

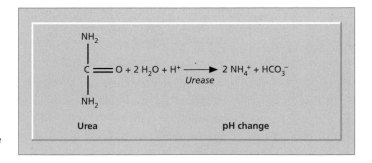

Fig. 4.1 The principle of the urease test.

species), and is more likely during therapy with antisecretory drugs and after gastric surgery. False-negative results may occur with low numbers of *H. pylori*. 'Homemade' kits for this test can be manufactured easily by the local pathology laboratory and cost only a few pence per test, but need to be validated.

High specificity and speed of result makes it a practical test

Rapid urease test provides an instant result, which can then be communicated to the clinician at the time the endoscopy report is furnished. Furthermore, because this test has a high specificity, *H. pylori* eradication therapy may be started (where indicated) without delay.

All of these biopsy-based methods may give false-negative results if only antral biopsies are taken within 1 week of taking proton pump inhibitors, antibiotics or bismuth. In such cases biopsies should also be taken from the body of the stomach.

Polymerase chain reaction

PCR has some drawbacks but is a useful research tool

Specific DNA sequences of *H. pylori* can be amplified by using pairs of specific oligonucleotides containing 10–15 bases (primers). The analysis of the amplification product allows the detection of *H. pylori* DNA. This is a highly specific and sensitive method for the detection of *H. pylori*, but because *H. pylori* DNA is being detected, non-viable bacteria may be found and, therefore, this technique has a limited role in confirming eradication of *H. pylori* after treatment. Another potential problem with PCR is contamination of specimens with DNA from previous patients. Biopsy forceps as well as endoscopes may be sources of contamination, even after standard cleaning and disinfection. One advantage of PCR is that it allows molecular typing of strains of *H. pylori*, and it is being used as a research tool.

Non-invasive tests available in primary care

Serology

This test is based on the detection of immunoglobulin G (IgG) antibodies specific to *H. pylori* in a serum sample. Several commercial *H. pylori* IgG enzyme-linked immunosorbent assay (ELISA) kits are available and are particularly useful for screening patients for *H. pylori* infection (Table 4.2). False-negative results may occur in children, the elderly and the

Table 4.2 'Near-patient' *H. pylori* IgG serology kits.

Test (manufacturer)	Sensitivity (%)	Specificity (%)
IgG ELISA Helisal Rapid Blood (Cortecs)	80–90	70–90
IgG ELISA Flexsure (SmithKline Diagnostics)	75	90
IgG LAT Pyloriset Dry (Orion)	95*	85*

* Manufacturer's data—no independent validation available.
LAT, latex agglutination test.

Serological tests are useful for screening patients

immunocompromised who have not raised an immunological response to the infection. All commercial serological kits need to be validated independently on the population to be studied by testing against a well-defined panel of sera, as the cut-off values provided by the manufacturer may not be valid. However, once validated in the population to be tested, IgG serology may be the best non-invasive technique to detect *H. pylori* infection, because it is simple to do, relatively specific and sensitive, and inexpensive. On the other hand, serology has a limited role in confirming eradication of *H. pylori* because it takes 6–12 months for the IgG titre to fall by 50% (usually taken as indicating eradication) or more of pre-treatment value.

Salivary tests for *H. pylori* are not as sensitive or specific as the serology-based tests and await further validation.

Some commercially available tests can be used in the GP surgery

Near-patient serological tests are now available commercially and are designed to provide an accurate and cost-effective diagnosis of *H. pylori* status for the primary care physician. These tests involve taking a sample of either capillary or whole blood from the subject, and provide a result within 15 minutes. However, the reported sensitivities and specificities of near-patient serological tests are not as high as the laboratory-based counterparts. Further development and validation are needed before they can be recommended (Table 4.2).

Urea breath tests (UBTs)

UBT uses either a radioactive or non-radioactive carbon label for urea

UBT is the most important non-invasive test for *H. pylori*, and may be used with either ^{13}C (non-radioactive) or ^{14}C (radioactive) isotopes. It is easy to do, safe, highly sensitive (95%) and specific (100%). The presence of labelled CO_2 in the

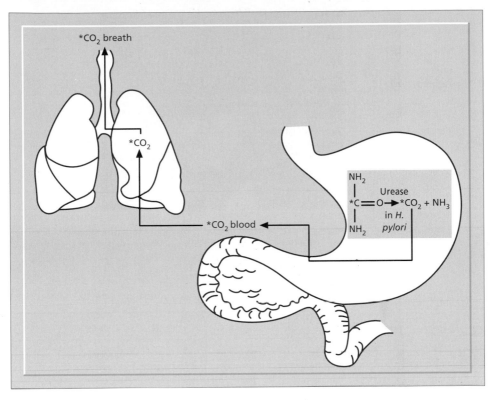

Fig. 4.2 The principle of the $^{13/14}$C-UBT. * = ^{13}C or ^{14}C. (Adapted with permission Mr Phil Johnson, Bureau of Stable Isotope Analysis, Brentford, UK.)

expired air indicates hydrolysis of urea and thus the presence of a urease-producing organism in the stomach (Fig. 4.2).

Method for ^{13}C-UBT

This test must be performed at least 4 hours after an endoscopy, or after a 6-hour fast. Three baseline samples of expired air are collected by the subject blowing through a straw, the tip of which is placed in the distal end of a test-tube (Fig. 4.3), until a blush of condensation appears on the container walls surrounding the end of the straw. The subject is given 100 ml of fatty (76% lipid) liquid test meal to delay gastric emptying. After 10 minutes ^{13}C-urea 100 mg in 50 ml of tap water is swallowed by the subject and distributed within the stomach by turning the patient to the left and right decubitus positions. Three breath samples are taken 30 minutes after the isotope. Breath samples are analysed by mass spectrometry

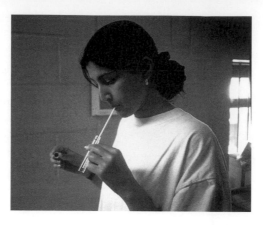

Fig. 4.3 Breath samples for the ^{13}C-UBT are collected by the subject blowing through a straw, the tip of which is placed at the distal end of a test-tube. (Reproduced with permission of Mr Phil Johnson, Bureau of Stable Isotope Analysis, Brentford, UK.)

Table 4.3 Performance of ^{13}C- and ^{14}C-UBT.

	^{13}C-UBT	^{14}C-UBT
Sensitivity	90–100%	90–100%
Specificity	90–100%	90–100%
Radioactive	No	Yes
Analysis	Isotope ratio mass spectrometry	Liquid scintillation counter
Advantages	Simple to do	Cheap
	Commercially available	Immediate results
Disadvantages	Cost (£25–£35)	Medical physics department regulations

Mass spectrometry or a scintillation counter is used to measure the labelled urea content of breath

(or in a scintillation counter if $^{14}CO_2$ is used). A positive result is defined as excess $\delta^{13}CO_2$ excretion greater than 5 ml^{-1}.

^{13}C-UBT versus ^{14}C-UBT

Overall performance of the two UBTs is similar (Table 4.3). The main difference between them is that ^{14}C-UBT is radioactive and is available only in units with a medical physics department, or a fully equipped research department. The amount of radiation exposure in the ^{14}C-UBT is negligible — about 10 tests give the same radiation dose as a chest radiograph — but it should be avoided in pregnant women and children. ^{13}C-UBT is more expensive because analysis is by isotope ratio mass spectrometry but, as the test materials are not radioactive, there are no contraindications to its use and no limit to the number of tests that can be done on any one individual.

False-negative results can occur if UBT is done within 1 week of taking proton pump inhibitors, bismuth or antibiotics, and after gastric surgery. False-positive results are possible if other urease-producing bacteria are present in the foregut, as may occur in patients with achlorhydria.

UBT is the best investigation for confirmation of H. *pylori* eradication, when it should be done at a minimum of 1 month after the end of treatment.

Further reading

Atherton JC, Spiller RC. The urea breath test for *Helicobacter pylori*. *Gut* 1994; **35**: 723–5.

Cutler AF, Havstad S, Ma CK *et al.* Accuracy of invasive and noninvasive tests to diagnose *Helicobacter pylori* infection. *Gastroenterology* 1995; **109**(1): 136–41.

Logan RPH, Polson RJ, Misiewicz JJ *et al.* Simplified single sample 13carbon urea breath test for *Helicobacter pylori*: comparison with histology, culture and ELISA serology. *Gut* 1991; **32**: 1461–4.

Peura DA. *Helicobacter pylori*: a diagnostic dilemma and a dilemma of diagnosis. *Gastroenterology* 1995; **109**(1): 313–14.

Sobala GM, Crabtree JE, Penrith JA *et al.* Screening dyspepsia by serology to *Helicobacter pylori*. *Lancet* 1991; **i**: 94–6.

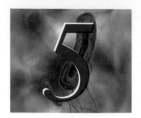

Treatment regimens for the eradication of *H. pylori*

Summary

- Monotherapy should not be used.
- Dual therapy with PPIs and amoxycillin or clarithromycin cures between 60 and 80% of *H. pylori*, but is highly dependent on patient's compliance with treatment.
- Classical triple therapy is a 2-week treatment, taking 11 tablets daily, with about 50% efficacy in metronidazole-resistant *H. pylori*.
- One-week low-dose triple therapy cures 85–95% of *H. pylori* with twice daily dosing, minimal side effects and is of proven efficacy in metronidazole-resistant strains.
- One-week quadruple therapy is effective, but requires motivated patients and is commonly associated with side effects.

Introduction

H. pylori eradication is defined as a negative *H. pylori* test 4 weeks or more after the end of treatment

The aim of treatment of *H. pylori* in any therapeutic context is eradication of the organism from the foregut. Eradication is defined as the presence of negative tests for *H. pylori* 4 weeks, or longer, after the end of antimicrobial therapy. Clearance or suppression of *H. pylori* may occur during treatment and tests done within 4 weeks of the end of medication may give false-negative results. This is because clearance, or suppression, is swiftly followed by recurrence of the original infection. The number and type of tests needed to establish eradication has not been universally agreed, but histology, bacterial culture of endoscopic biopsies, the CLO™ test or the ^{13}C- or ^{14}C-urea breath tests are used singly, or in various combinations. Serology can also be used for this purpose, but as the fall in *H. pylori*-specific antibody titres takes more than 6 months to develop, it has not been employed widely in monitoring the effects of therapy. The specificity and sensitivity of these tests have been established variously in separate studies and is reviewed in Chapter 4. The best test to use in order to confirm

The urea breath test is the
most clinically useful test
for confirmation of
treatment outcome

successful outcome of anti-*H. pylori* treatment in clinical practice is the urea breath test.

Antibacterial treatment of *H. pylori* is difficult because of the habitat occupied by the organism below the layer of mucus adherent to the gastric mucosa. Access of antimicrobial agents to this site is limited from the lumen of the stomach and also from the gastric blood supply.

Another adverse factor is the resistance of *Helicobacter* to antimicrobial agents, especially to nitroimidazoles (metronidazole and tinidazole), which develops rapidly during therapy, or pre-exists in the community, especially among ethnic minorities. The high prevalence of *H. pylori* strains resistant to metronidazole because of previous usage of this agent by Caucasian women, or by subjects of either gender in the developing world, has been well documented.

Metronidazole resistance
is common, and can
develop during therapy or
pre-exist due to previous
use

These factors have led to the concurrent use of multiple agents, as exemplified by dual, triple or quadruple therapy regimens. Although these are effective, the somewhat complex treatment schedules and unwanted effects of the drugs lessen compliance and thus their efficacy. Resistance to antibiotics other than nitroimidazoles, for example to clarithromycin, can also develop, but is much rarer. The problem of resistance is very important; it readily occurs with monotherapy which therefore should never be used for *Helicobacter*.

Resistance frequently
occurs with monotherapy

The ideal therapy for *H. pylori* eradication should be simple, safe, free from side effects, with 100% efficacy and low cost. The ideal treatment regimen has not been defined yet and it is not possible currently to make definite recommendations for the optimal treatment schedule. The problem is compounded by the plethora of small-scale therapeutic trials that have flooded the literature. Many, if not most, of the existing studies are not double blind, and there are virtually no studies comparing two treatment regimens concurrently in the same population of patients. Details of doses, frequency of dosing and duration of treatment vary between the trials, limiting the scope for meta-analysis.

Meta-analysis is
complicated by the degree
of variation between trials

The treatment for *H. pylori* should not be given lightly and only after due consideration of the clinical diagnosis and the proper indications for eradication. Prescribing various combinations of bismuth, antibiotics and acid suppressants with variable dosages and timings for patients with 'dyspepsia' must not be done. It may do harm in the form of side effects, including very occasionally pseudomembranous colitis, and the emergence of resistant organisms.

Anti-Helicobacter
treatment should only be
given for specific
indications

Eradication regimens are discussed under the heading of mono, dual, triple and quadruple therapy, depending on the number of antimicrobial agents used concurrently in the treatment. Eradication percentages are reported regardless of the underlying diagnoses. This is because many studies have recruited non-uniform populations (for example, mixtures of patients with duodenal ulcer and functional dyspepsia). Moreover, there is at present insufficient knowledge of the response to treatment of strains of *H. pylori* associated with peptic ulcer, as compared with those causing gastritis only, to justify separate analyses.

Antibiotic bioavailability

In vitro tests of bacterial sensitivity may not predict sensitivity *in vitro*

The *in vitro* susceptibility of *H. pylori* to an antibiotic does not necessarily predict its *in vivo* effectiveness. Effectiveness of an antimicrobial agent may be modified as a result of the acid environment of the stomach decreasing the effectiveness of some agents. In other cases concentrations achieved in the gastric pits are low and there may be a failure to eradicate the bacterium in the fundus. The concentrations and activity of drugs in the gastric mucosa, mucus and crypts may be affected by drug formulation and route of administration. For example, after oral administration of amoxycillin the highest tissue concentrations are found in the antrum and the lowest in the fundus. Studies on the effect of the timing of amoxycillin in relationship to meals on eradication of *H. pylori* have shown that pre-prandial dosing with amoxycillin *capsules* was no more effective than post-prandial. On the other hand, pre-prandial dosing with amoxycillin *suspension* was more effective than post-prandial when given in combination with once daily omeprazole, suggesting that a systemic effect of amoxycillin is important for eradication of *H. pylori*. By contrast, the formulation of tripotassium dicitrato bismuthate as either tablets or liquid, appears to make little difference to *H. pylori* eradication.

Modes of action of anti-*H. pylori* agents

Bismuth

The mechanism by which bismuth salts act on *H. pylori* is imperfectly understood. Transmucosal penetration of bismuth particles in the antrum has been observed after oral dosing with colloidal bismuth subcitrate (CBS), but not with bismuth subsalicylate (BSS). CBS has been shown to block adhesion of *H. pylori* to epithelial cells, to accumulate along bacterial membranes, to form protective complexes with glycoproteins and to stimulate mucosal bicarbonate secretion.

The mechanism of action of bismuth is not fully understood

Proton pump inhibitors (PPIs)

In vitro studies have shown that omeprazole, lansoprazole and pantoprazole have a bacteriostatic effect on *H. pylori*. The MIC_{90} of lansoprazole is fourfold lower than omeprazole (6.25 µg ml^{-1} versus 25 µg ml^{-1}), but the *in vivo* significance of this finding is uncertain. The mechanism of the bacteriostatic effect is unclear, but covalent binding of the activated drugs to thiol groups on the *H. pylori* membrane may occur. Alternatively, the PPIs may interfere with energy production by the bacterium; adenosine triphosphatase (ATPase) activity along the cell membrane of *H. pylori* has been reported and its activity was shown to be inhibited by PPIs in an acid environment. All three PPIs lead to a transient decrease in the antral *H. pylori* density during therapy, although the fundal bacterial density may be increased, leading to fundal gastritis. This may be important when considering maintenance treatment with PPIs for gastro-oesophageal reflux disease in patients colonised with *H. pylori*, because fundal gastritis may occur and, with time, gastric atrophy (and intestinal metaplasia). The latter is a recognised risk factor for the development of carcinoma. In this group of patients it may be appropriate to eradicate *H. pylori* before starting long-term PPI treatment.

PPIs have a bacteriostatic effect, possibly by binding covalently to the *H. pylori* membrane

Eradication is considered before long-term PPI treatment in *H. pylori*-positive patients

Clarithromycin

Clarithromycin is one of the most active antimicrobial agents against *H. pylori in vitro*, with a MIC_{90} of 0.03 µg ml^{-1} (10 times lower than erythromycin). Clarithromycin is readily absorbed and attains high serum and tissue concentrations after oral dosing. It is metabolised to a pharmacologically active metabolite, 14-hydroxy-clarithromycin, which possesses activity against *H. pylori*. At pH 5.5, attainable with PPIs, clarithromycin is the most active antimicrobial agent (MIC_{90} 0.25 µg ml^{-1}). The administration of clarithromycin with omeprazole increases plasma concentrations of clarithromycin and 14-hydroxy-clarithromycin.

The high antimicrobial activity of clarithromycin is enhanced by PPIs

Histamine H_2 receptor antagonists (H_2RAs)

H_2RAs have no intrinsic or *in vivo* activity on *H. pylori*.

H. pylori eradication regimens

All current treatments for eradication of *H. pylori* are associated with side effects and their type and frequency are indicated in Tables 5.1–5.6.

Monotherapy

Monotherapy with antibiotics is not recommended

Single agents are generally ineffective or poorly effective in eradicating *H. pylori* and are therefore discussed only briefly. Eradication with single antibiotics ranges from 0 to 54%, the most effective being clarithromycin, where 500 mg q.d.s. for 2 weeks was reported to produce 54% *H. pylori* eradication. Amoxycillin (up to $6\,g\,day^{-1}$), cephalosporins and ciprofloxacin are ineffective on their own. Monotherapy with any antibiotic is proscribed, not only because it is ineffective, but because it is also liable to produce resistant organisms.

Despite the demonstration of an *in vitro* anti-*H. pylori* effect of PPIs, which is greatest with lansoprazole, none of the PPIs alone possesses any useful eradicating properties *in vivo*.

Bismuth compounds suppress but do not eradicate *H. pylori*

Bismuth compounds suppress *H. pylori*, which explains, at least in part, the decreased incidence of relapse reported after bismuth monotherapy before the discovery of *H. pylori*. Ranitidine bismuth citrate (RBC) used as monotherapy suppresses, but does not eradicate *H. pylori*.

Dual therapy

Antibiotics

The combination of two antimicrobial agents, for example tinidazole and amoxycillin, does not lead to reliable *H. pylori* eradication.

H_2RAs with antibiotics

Ranitidine plus an antibiotic has some success as an eradication therapy

There has been limited success with H_2RAs in combination with a single antibiotic for eradication of *H. pylori*. High-dose ranitidine (300 mg b.d.) has been co-prescribed with either amoxycillin or clarithromycin for 2 weeks with limited success, with *H. pylori* eradication in up to 60% of patients.

Bismuth with antibiotics

CBS, in combination with metronidazole has been reported to eradicate *H. pylori* in up to 85% of patients. However, the number of patients per study has been small, drug regimens are variable between studies and, most importantly, most of the studies have selected subjects colonised with metronidazole-sensitive strains (MSS) for the whole, or for most of the study population. RBC (400–800 mg b.d.) has been tried in combination with either amoxycillin (500 mg q.d.s.) or clarithromycin (250 mg q.d.s.) for 14 days, with *H. pylori* eradication of about 65% with amoxycillin, but with clarithromycin the figures become 83% with RBC 400 mg b.d. and 71% with RBC 800 mg b.d. These results are calculated on an intention-to-treat ('worst case scenario') basis (Tables 5.1 & 5.2). These regimens, despite involving only two agents,

RBC has a higher eradication with clarithromycin than with amoxycillin

Table 5.1 Dual therapy with amoxycillin.

	Dual therapy	
	omeprazole amoxycillin	RBC amoxycillin
Dosing	20–40 mg b.d. 500 mg q.d.s. or 1 g b.d.	400–800 mg b.d. 500 mg q.d.s.
Duration	2 weeks	2 weeks
H. pylori eradication	50–85%	65%
Side effects	Common: diarrhoea	Common: diarrhoea

Table 5.2 Dual therapy with clarithromycin.

	Dual therapy	
	omeprazole clarithromycin	RBC clarithromycin
Dosing	40 mg o.d. 500 mg t.d.s.	400 mg b.d. 250 mg q.d.s.
Duration	2 weeks	2 weeks
H. pylori eradication	60–80%	80%
Side effects	Common: taste disturbances, diarrhoea	Common: taste disturbances, diarrhoea

require motivated patients to take antimicrobial agents four times daily for 2 weeks.

PPIs *with clarithromycin* (Table 5.2)

Inhibition of acid secretion, for example with PPIs, raises the intragastric pH to 5.0 or higher, and significantly decreases the MIC_{90} of some antibiotics (amoxycillin and clarithromycin) and so makes them more effective. The combination of various dosages and durations of PPIs (such as omeprazole and increasingly lansoprazole) and clarithromycin for *H. pylori* eradication have been studied. Initial studies used 2 weeks' treatment, but there are some preliminary reports suggesting that 7 days' therapy with high-dose omeprazole (40 mg b.d.) and clarithromycin (500 mg b.d.) may be as effective, with around 80% *H. pylori* eradication. There are some indications that the frequency of dosing and total dose of clarithromycin may be important. Thus, clarithromycin (500 mg) given twice daily in combination with omeprazole 40 mg was apparently less effective, with eradication reported as 56%, compared with 63–81% on clarithromycin (500 mg) three times daily. Side effects occur in about 50% of patients treated with clarithromycin and omeprazole and become more common as the dose and frequency of clarithromycin increase, the most common being taste disturbance. Clarithromycin is a relatively expensive antimicrobial agent. A 2-week combination of omeprazole 40 mg o.d. and clarithromycin 500 mg t.d.s. costs about £90, which is considerably more than most other regimens (£15–£30).

> Inhibition of acid secretion increases efficacy of some antibiotics

> A side effect of clarithromycin is taste disturbance

PPIs *and amoxycillin* (see Table 5.1)

Most of the work dealing with dual therapy using PPIs, such as omeprazole, and amoxycillin is published as abstracts. The results suggest that the daily dose of amoxycillin should be at least 2 g; the frequency of administration appears to be less important than the compliance with the treatment regimen. In combination with amoxycillin, omeprazole is more effective when given twice daily and at higher than normal doses. Thus, eradication with omeprazole 20 mg or 40 mg o.d. with amoxycillin 2 g daily for 2 weeks varies between 0 and 28%, but on omeprazole 20–40 mg b.d. in combination with amoxycillin 1 g b.d. (or 500 mg q.d.s.) for 2 weeks' eradication was 50–90%. It is not known whether these interesting observations were due to more effective control of intragastric acidity,

> This combination requires a high dose of omeprazole

Table 5.3 Non-PPI triple therapy combinations with amoxycillin and metronidazole.

	Triple therapy	
	CBS amoxycillin metronidazole	ranitidine amoxycillin metronidazole
Dosing	120 mg q.d.s. 500 mg q.d.s. 200–400 mg q.d.s.	300 mg o.d. 750 mg t.d.s. 500 mg t.d.s.
Duration	2 weeks	12 days
H. pylori eradication	60–90%	90%
Side effects	Common: diarrhoea, nausea	Common: diarrhoea, nausea

or to some intrinsic property of omeprazole affecting *H. pylori*, or to some other mechanism. There is a paucity of data on pantoprazole, or lansoprazole in combination with amoxycillin, but preliminary studies suggest that these newer PPIs are as effective as omeprazole.

Triple therapy

Classical triple therapy (Table 5.3)

The most thoroughly studied *H. pylori* eradication regimen consists of CBS, metronidazole and either amoxycillin or tetracycline. There are wide variations in the dosage and treatment schedules used in classical triple therapy regimens, with eradication results varying from 30 to 95%. It is difficult to account for these differences, except by invoking the customary factors of dissimilarities in patient populations, incidence of metronidazole resistance, degrees of compliance with the treatment and the like. The effect of duration of therapy on eradication results has not been studied systematically in comparable populations and clinical settings. Thus, although the best results were recorded in a trial lasting 30 days, broadly comparable data are reported with shorter treatments. On the other hand, it has to be borne in mind that classical triple therapy given for less than 7 days has not been successful. It can be tentatively concluded that triple therapy given for longer than 14 days appears to give no further therapeutic advantage. Comparison of tetracycline with amoxycillin-based triple therapies does not show any significant advantage in terms of eradication for one

Eradication results vary between 30 and 95%

Metronidazole-resistant
H. pylori is less responsive
to classical triple therapy

over the other. Triple therapy with either amoxycillin or tetra-cycline is not very effective for eradication of metronidazole-resistant *H. pylori*, with most eradication results falling between 33 and 63% in this group of patients.

Ampicillin, oxacillin, clarithromycin, ofloxacin, ciproflox-acin and doxycycline have been tried in place of amoxycillin or tetracycline, with less therapeutic success.

Bismuth plus antibiotic plus PPI

Eradication with these regimens varies from 15 to 90%. Preliminary data from a pilot study using a 1-week regimen consisting of CBS 240 mg b.d., clarithromycin 500 mg t.d.s. and omeprazole 20 mg b.d. reported over 90% *H. pylori* eradication.

Non-bismuth-based triple therapy regimens (Table 5.3)

Drug regimens that do not include bismuth are of particular interest in the context of *H. pylori* eradication. This is because bismuth is said to act on the gastric mucosa through several mechanisms, apart from its anti-*H. pylori* capability. Regimens without bismuth therefore show their therapeutic potential more precisely through the elimination of *H. pylori*, rather than through some other pharmacological effect.

Ranitidine with
metronidazole and
amoxycillin is useful

Ranitidine 300 mg o.d. combined with metronidazole 500 mg t.d.s. and amoxycillin 750 mg t.d.s. for 12 days was shown to eradicate around 90% of *H. pylori*. However, this regimen is far less effective against metronidazole-resistant strains, where eradication is around 50%.

PPI-based triple therapy regimens (Table 5.4)

The combination of a PPI plus clarithromycin and a nitroimi-dazole (metronidazole or tinidazole) taken twice daily for 1 week has been a very successful regimen in the studies reported so far, with *H. pylori* eradication consistently around 90%. There is no therapeutic advantage in increasing the dose of clarithromycin above 500 mg daily, or metronidazole above 800 mg daily, but continuing treatment for more than 7 days might be better—this needs confirmation at present. These low-dose, triple therapy regimens appear to be associated with few side effects; nausea and diarrhoea being the most common. Amoxycillin has been tried in place of clarithromycin to

A short treatment regimen
with few side effects

Table 5.4 Low-dose, 1-week triple therapy regimens.

	Triple therapy		
	lansoprazole/omeprazole clarithromycin metronidazole	lansoprazole/omeprazole amoxycillin metronidazole	lansoprazole/omeprazole amoxycillin clarithromycin
Dosing	30 mg or 20 mg b.d. 250 mg b.d. 400 mg b.d.	30 mg or 40 mg o.d. 500 mg t.d.s. 400 mg t.d.s.	30 mg or 20 mg b.d. 1 g b.d. 250 mg b.d.
Duration	7 days	7 days	7 days
H. pylori eradication	>90%	85–90%	85–90%
Side effects	Minimal: nausea	Common: diarrhoea, nausea	Common: diarrhoea, nausea

Table 5.5 Quadruple therapy.

	omeprazole CBS tetracycline metronidazole
Dosing	20 mg o.d.–b.d. 120 mg q.d.s. 500 mg q.d.s. 400–500 mg q.d.s./t.d.s.
Duration	7 days
H. pylori eradication	86–98%
Side effects	Common: diarrhoea, nausea

decrease costs and the development of widespread clarithromycin resistance, with similar but more variable results.

The combination of lansoprazole 30 mg o.d. (or omeprazole 40 mg o.d.), amoxycillin 500 mg t.d.s. and metronidazole 400 mg t.d.s. for 1 week is an effective triple therapy, with *H. pylori* eradicated in around 90% of the patients, but more impressive was the 75–80% eradication of metronidazole-resistant *H. pylori*.

Quadruple therapy (Table 5.5)

Compliance becomes a problem the more complex the regimen

Quadruple therapy for *H. pylori* eradication must entail more compliance problems and side effects than the simpler regimens. Despite this, 98% *H. pylori* eradication has been reported using a 1-week combination of omeprazole (20 mg b.d.—given for a total of 10 days), CBS (120 mg q.d.s.), tetra-

Table 5.6 Therapies proven against metronidazole-resistant *H. pylori* strains.

	Therapy		
	lansoprazole amoxicillin clarithromycin	omeprazole amoxicillin metronidazole	omeprazole CBS tetracycline metronidazole
Dosing	30 mg b.d. 1 g b.d. 250 mg b.d.	40 mg o.d. 500 mg t.d.s. 400 mg t.d.s.	20 mg o.d. 120 mg q.d.s. 500 mg q.d.s. 400 mg q.d.s.
Duration	1 week	1 week	1 week
H. pylori eradication	>90%	>80%	90%
Side effects	Uncommon: nausea, diarrhoea	Common: nausea, diarrhoea	Common: nausea, diarrhoea

cycline (500 mg q.d.s.) and metronidazole (500 mg t.d.s.). Compliance was remarkably high in this well-performed study, and all patients were followed up. Only 7.7% of the *H. pylori* pre-treatment isolates were metronidazole resistant, and this may account for the very high eradication reported.

Metronidazole-resistant organisms (Table 5.6)

Metronidazole-resistant *H. pylori* are more difficult to eradicate and Table 5.6 outlines therapies that have been shown to be effective in these cases. Ideally, a regimen not containing a nitroimidazole should be used, such as lansoprazole (or omeprazole), amoxicillin and clarithromycin (Table 5.6), with 90% *H. pylori* eradication in patients with pre-treatment metronidazole-resistant strains of *H. pylori*. Classical triple therapy using bismuth and metronidazole with either amoxicillin or tetracycline, is not very effective for eradication of metronidazole-resistant *H. pylori*, and is successful in only 50% of cases. Similar results are obtained with ranitidine in combination with amoxicillin and metronidazole. However, the 1-week, low-dose triple therapies containing lansoprazole, clarithromycin and metronidazole have been reported to be almost as effective in the presence of pre-treatment metronidazole-resistant strains of *H. pylori*, with *H. pylori* eradication of about 80%. Another effective treatment for metronidazole-resistant strains is quadruple therapy involving omeprazole, bismuth, tetracycline and metronidazole, with

Nitroimidazoles should not be included in this regimen

Omeprazole, bismuth,
tetracycline and
metronidazole are more
than 90% successful

more than 90% success. Less demanding, and almost as effective triple therapy regimens are shown in Table 5.6. Culture of *H. pylori* from endoscopic biopsies after failure of apparently adequate eradication treatment with good compliance may be needed to appraise the situation with sensitivity tests and prescribe the most appropriate drug combination. In some cases the bacterium defeats all attempts at eradication and definitive treatment may have to be abandoned; fortunately, such instances are rare.

Conclusion

There are thus many different regimens available for the eradication of *H. pylori*. As there are still only a few published large controlled trials, and as comparative trials are conspicuous by their absence, it is difficult to give firm recommendations as to which is the best regimen to use. Indeed, it is possible that the results of triple or quadruple therapies are similar, and that their efficacy may depend more on other factors, such as ease of compliance, freedom from side effects and effectiveness against metronidazole-resistant strains of *H. pylori*. Counselling of the patient before treatment is started is important. Cost is also a consideration, but as drugs are priced differently in different purchasing schemes, prices have not been detailed here. In general, regimens providing three therapeutic agents are preferred. High prevalence of metronidazole-resistant strains in the community (e.g. immigrants from the emergent countries), may lead to preference for non-metronidazole treatment regimens.

Little comparative data
exist on eradication
regimens

Further reading

Bazzoli F, Zagari RM, Fossi S *et al.* Short-term low-dose triple therapy for the eradication of *Helicobacter pylori. Eur J Gastroenterol Hepatol* 1994; **6**: 773–7.

Bell GD, Powell KU, Burridge SM *et al. Helicobacter pylori* eradication: efficacy and side effect profile of a combination of omeprazole, amoxycillin and metronidazole compared with four alternative regimens. *Quatern J Med* 1993; **86**: 743–50.

Harris AW, Misiewicz JJ. Eradication of *Helicobacter pylori.* In: Calam J, ed. *Baillière's Clinical Gastroenterology*: Helicobacter pylori *Infection*. London, UK: Baillière Tindall, 1995; **9**(3): 583–613.

Hentschel E, Brandstatter G, Dragosics B *et al.* Effect of ranitidine and amoxycillin plus metronidazole on the eradication of *Helicobacter pylori* and the recurrence of duodenal ulcer. *N Engl J Med* 1993; **328**: 308–12.

Labenz J, Gyenes E, Ruhi GH *et al.* Amoxycillin plus omeprazole versus triple therapy for eradication of *Helicobacter pylori* in duodenal ulcer disease: a prospective randomized and controlled study. *Gut* 1993; **34**: 1167–70.

Lind T, Veldhuyzen van Zanten SJO, Unge P *et al.* The MACH 1 study: optimal one-week treatment for *H. pylori* defined? *Gut* 1995; **37** (Suppl. 1): A4.

Misiewicz JJ, Harris AW, Bardham KD *et al.* One week low-dose triple therapy for eradication of *H. pylori*: a large multicentre, randomised trial. *Gut* 1996; **38** (Suppl. 1): A1.

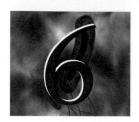

Indications for eradication of *H. pylori*

Summary

• 90–95% of duodenal and gastric ulcers not associated with NSAIDs are caused by *H. pylori*.
• Eradication of *H. pylori* heals the ulcer and decreases relapse.
• No convincing evidence for an association between functional dyspepsia and *H. pylori*.
• *H. pylori* is associated with a two- to sixfold increase in risk of developing gastric cancer, but there are no overall indications for eradication, unless risk factors exist.
• *H. pylori* may be associated with an increased risk of developing coronary heart disease, but the evidence is preliminary and coronary heart disease is not an indication for treatment.
• Eradication of *H. pylori* has resulted in regression of the rare low-grade B-cell gastric lymphoma of mucosa-associated lymphoid tissue (MALT) and Ménétrier's disease.

Peptic ulcer disease

Relapse rate in DU and GU patients is reduced by *H. pylori* eradication

It is now generally agreed that *H. pylori* is the cause of virtually all duodenal (DU) and chronic benign gastric ulcer (GU) disease that is not associated with NSAIDs. More than 95% of patients with DU are colonised with *H. pylori* (Fig. 6.1) and eradication of this infection leads to a dramatic decrease in the relapse rate from 80% after healing of the ulcer with other agents, to less than 5% each year. About 90% of patients with chronic benign non-NSAID GU are colonised with *H. pylori*, and eradication of this bacterium not only heals the ulcer, but prevents relapse (Table 6.1).

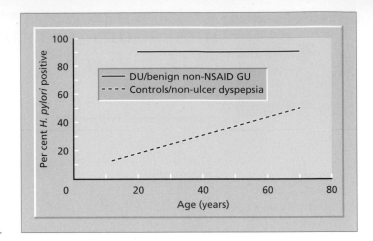

Fig. 6.1 Incidence of *H. pylori* in clinical conditions.

Table 6.1 Guidelines for *H. pylori* eradication.

Diagnosis	*H. pylori* status	Eradication treatment
Asymptomatic	Negative	No
	Positive	No
Functional dyspepsia	Negative	No
	Positive	No
Duodenal ulcer	Negative	No
	Positive	Yes
Gastric ulcer	Negative	No
	Positive	Yes
Strong family history of gastric cancer*	Negative	No
	Positive	Yes

* See p. 55.

Duodenal ulcer

Diagnosis

Endoscopic diagnosis of non-NSAID DU is sufficient to initiate eradication therapy

On the simplest level, a patient with well-documented endo-scopically diagnosed DU (Plate 6.1, facing p. 26) who is not taking ulcerogenic drugs (such as NSAIDs) can be assumed to be colonised with *H. pylori* and eradication treatment can be prescribed without any further tests. If there is any doubt, such as a possible ulcer crater seen on barium meal, endoscopic con-firmation should be sought before prescribing the treatment. Some clinicians may prefer to establish *Helicobacter* status before starting eradication therapy. This can be done non-invasively using serology or urea breath test (UBT), or at

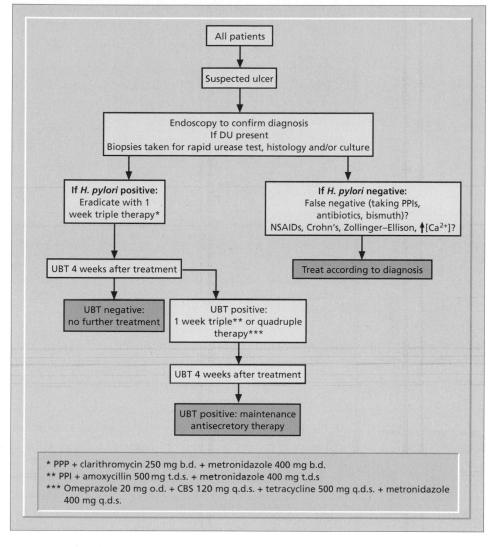

Fig. 6.2 Management plan for DU. PPI, proton pump inhibitor.

Inside figure:

All patients

Suspected ulcer

Endoscopy to confirm diagnosis
If DU present
Biopsies taken for rapid urease test, histology and/or culture

If *H. pylori* positive:
Eradicate with 1
week triple therapy*

If *H. pylori* negative:
False negative (taking PPIs,
antibiotics, bismuth)?
NSAIDs, Crohn's, Zollinger–Ellison, $\uparrow[Ca^{2+}]$?

UBT 4 weeks after treatment

Treat according to diagnosis

UBT negative:
no further treatment

UBT positive:
1 week triple** or quadruple
therapy***

UBT 4 weeks after treatment

UBT positive: maintenance
antisecretory therapy

* PPP + clarithromycin 250 mg b.d. + metronidazole 400 mg b.d.
** PPI + amoxycillin 500 mg t.d.s. + metronidazole 400 mg t.d.s
*** Omeprazole 20 mg o.d. + CBS 120 mg q.d.s. + tetracycline 500 mg q.d.s. + metronidazole
400 mg q.d.s.

---

endoscopy with biopsies for rapid urease test, histology or bacterial culture (see Chapter 4). A management plan for *H. pylori*-positive and -negative DU patients is outlined in Fig. 6.2.

All patients with DU and *H. pylori* infection should be treated with *H. pylori* eradication therapy, regardless of whether they are seen at the initial presentation of the disease, or at a recurrence. Symptom-free patients on long-term (maintenance) treatment with H_2 receptor antagonists, or proton pump inhibitors, should also be given eradication treatment. Success-

Eradication therapy saves on the cost of long-term antisecretory treatment

---

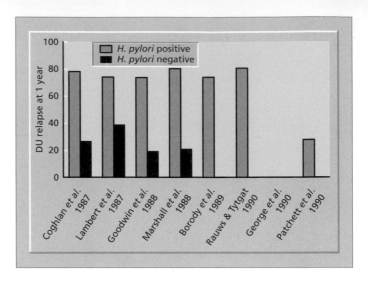

Fig. 6.3 DU relapse related to post-treatment *H. pylori* status. For details see Rauws BAJ, Tytgat GNJ. *Helicobacter pylori* in duodenal and gastric ulcer disease. *Baillière's Clin Gastroenterol* 1995; **9**(3): 529–47.

ful eradication will make further maintenance therapy unnecessary, with significant savings of prescribing costs (Fig. 6.3).

After treatment

DU heal quickly and completely after eradication of *H. pylori*, and many clinicians believe that a separate healing course of antisecretory treatment is unnecessary. Unless complicating features (such as recent haemorrhage or perforation) are present, repeat endoscopy after treatment of a DU is unnecessary. It can be argued that after eradication treatment it is reasonable to await clinical outcome, rather than to test formally for the absence or presence of the bacterium. However, we feel that it is preferable to confirm the success, or otherwise, of therapy, as symptoms may not be abolished completely by eradication of *H. pylori* and unless the result of the therapy is known, further management may not be clear. Another way is to await the clinical outcome and if there are residual symptoms, tests for *H. pylori* should be done then.

Confirm the outcome with a *H. pylori* test

Tests to confirm successful eradication of *H. pylori* should be performed no sooner than 28 days after the end of eradication treatment, because suppression of *H. pylori* immediately after treatment may lead to a false-negative test result. Furthermore, proton pump inhibitors, bismuth and antibiotics may interfere with the sensitivity of the diagnostic methods used to determine *H. pylori* status, and thus must be avoided for the 2 weeks before the test (see Chapter 4). The ^{13}C-UBT is the best test for confirmation of eradication of *H. pylori*, being safe, accurate and non-invasive. Serology will not produce interpretable results in under 6 months after the end of therapy, as the antibody titre falls slowly after eradication.

Complications of DU, such as bleeding and perforation, are associated with high morbidity and mortality. There is some evidence that eradication of *H. pylori* in patients with bleeding DU may prevent recurrence of bleeding from the ulcer. However, until prospective randomised trials confirm these preliminary studies it is prudent to start maintenance antisecretory treatment even before confirming successful eradication of *H. pylori* in these high-risk patients. By contrast, there is no evidence that eradication of *H. pylori* prevents re-perforation of DU. Thus, patients with a history of perforated DU should be offered eradication treatment (if colonised by *H. pylori*, and only about 50% will be), but also started immediately on maintenance antisecretory treatment in the usual way.

In about 5% of initially *H. pylori*-positive patients with DU the ulcer may recur after successful eradication of the bacterium, but in the absence of re-infection with *H. pylori* or NSAID consumption. In these individuals it is important to exclude other ulcerogenic drug ingestions, Zollinger–Ellison syndrome, Crohn's disease, hypercalcaemia, sarcoidosis or ectopic pancreatic tissue in the duodenal bulb. In the absence of these conditions, there is evidence to suggest that these patients with DU have increased parietal cell mass and high gastric acid output; possibly as an inherited characteristic. In this small subgroup of patients with DU, maintenance antisecretory treatment is needed to prevent further ulcer relapse.

If patients have a symptomatic relapse, but without DU recurrence after proven eradication of *H. pylori*, further investigations may be necessary to exclude gastro-oesophageal reflux disease (GORD) and gall stones by barium swallow and ultrasound scan, respectively. Indeed, there are reports that the frequency of symptomatic GORD increases after eradication of *H. pylori* in patients with previous DU, possibly as a result of dietary changes and weight gain. Furthermore, the abdominal symptoms that had been assumed to be due to DU disease may persist after eradication of *H. pylori* and actually be related to functional dyspepsia, or irritable bowel syndrome

Patients with a history of bleeding or perforation need antisecretory therapy in addition to anti-H. pylori treatment

In a small proportion of patients non-H. pylori-related DU recurrence may be seen

Some studies have found an increased risk of GORD after eradication

(see below). In this case dietary modifications, prokinetic and antispasmodic drugs may be indicated.

Gastric ulcer

Diagnosis

The management of GU differs from that of DU, the main point of difference being the need to exclude the presence of malignancy in an apparently benign GU (Fig. 6.4). This is done by multiple endoscopic targeted biopsies before and after GU healing. It is advisable to re-endoscope GU patients some 8–12 weeks after treatment to confirm healing and obtain further biopsies; *H. pylori* status can be ascertained at the same time by histology and/or the CLO™ test (see Chapter 4).

Management of GU involves the exclusion of malignancy

Treatment

Patients with *H. pylori* infection and GU should be offered eradication therapy. Eradication of *H. pylori* leads to healing of the ulcer and very significantly decreases the incidence of relapse of GU. At present the effect of eradication of *H. pylori* on GU complications is unknown and maintenance antisecretory treatment should be started immediately in those patients with GU who have a history of haemorrhage or perforation. *H. pylori* eradication and GU healing should be confirmed by endoscopy at 8–12 weeks after the end of treatment.

Endoscopy should confirm success 8–12 weeks after treatment

Ulcers associated with NSAID treatment

The incidence of *H. pylori* infection in patients with NSAID-associated ulceration is similar to that of the general population in the same age groups. The clinical benefit, if any, of *H. pylori* eradication in *H. pylori*-positive patients with NSAID-induced GU or DU is unclear at present, but there is some preliminary data which suggest that NSAID-induced mucosal damage is decreased in the absence of *H. pylori*. There thus appears to be some justification in offering *H. pylori* eradication to a patient with a DU or GU who is on NSAIDs and who is colonised by the bacterium. Eradication would not obviate the need for other therapy for the ulcer and the usual rules for minimising NSAID damage still apply. Treatment with NSAIDs, or aspirin, should not alter the antimicrobial regimen, but these drugs should be discontinued whenever possible.

NSAID-induced mucosal damage may be decreased in the absence of *H. pylori*

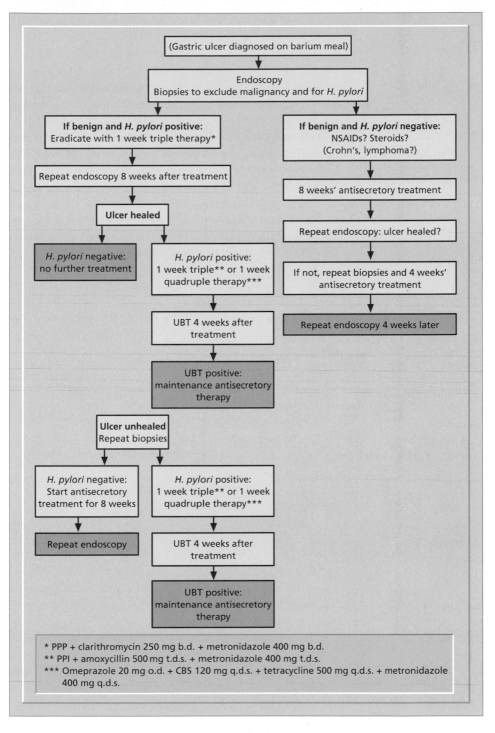

Fig. 6.4 Management plan for GU.

Functional (non-ulcer) dyspepsia

At present there is no convincing evidence for an association between *H. pylori* infection and functional dyspepsia. The prevalence of *H. pylori* infection is no higher in patients with functional dyspepsia than in the general population. Although a subset of patients with functional dyspepsia (ulcer-like dyspepsia) may exist in whom symptoms are related to the presence of *H. pylori*, there is so far little evidence showing clear clinical benefit after eradication of *H. pylori*. Until the results of large, well-controlled trials are available, there is at present no indication for eradication of *H. pylori* in functional dyspepsia. Patients with this condition continue to be managed on the usual lines (Fig. 6.5).

H. pylori eradication is not indicated for functional dyspepsia

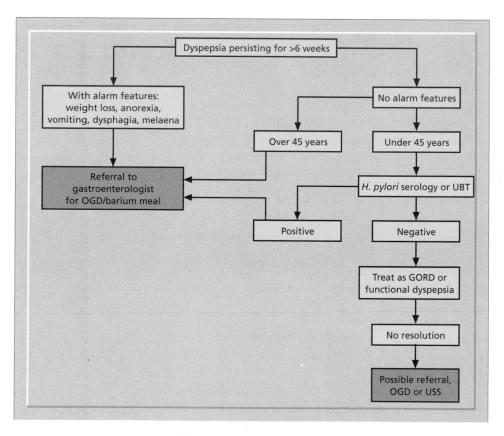

Fig. 6.5 Management plan for dyspepsia. OGD, oesophago-gastroduodenoscopy; USS, abdominal ultrasound scan.

Screening for *H. pylori* before endoscopy

Endoscopy workloads are ever-increasing and in many parts of the country there are long waiting lists for this expensive procedure. Several studies have explored the possibility of using screening (usually by serology, but also by UBT) before referring the patient for gastroscopy. The principle of this type of screening hinges on the assumption that in the younger patient (45 years or younger) with symptoms suggesting DU (not GORD), who is not on ulcerogenic drugs and otherwise in good health, gastric malignancy, lymphoma or GU are extremely unlikely. Moreover, if the patient is *H. pylori* negative, DU is virtually excluded in such circumstances (see Fig. 6.2).

H. pylori screening without endoscopy is acceptable for younger patients

Several studies have shown that if *H. pylori*-negative patients fulfilling the above criteria are not endoscoped, serious lesions would not be missed, although a few cases of oesophagitis would have escaped diagnosis. *Helicobacter* tests in a young patient with ulcer-like dyspepsia thus obviate the need for endoscopic referral. If the patient tests negative he/she is treated with antacids, promotility drugs, or possibly with acid suppressive therapy, as indicated clinically. If this course of management is adopted, the patient should be followed up to check progress. Should there be deterioration in general health, anorexia, weight loss, vomiting or severe pain unresponsive to treatment, then further investigations must be done. This approach is safe, provided the doctor exercises clinical judgement, follows the patient up and correctly interprets the patient's clinical state.

Gastric cancer

A number of large-scale prospective and retrospective epidemiological studies have reported an association between *H. pylori* and gastric cancer. A multicentre study involving over 3000 subjects in 13 countries found a significant positive correlation between regional variations in gastric cancer mortality and differences in the seroprevalence of *H. pylori* infection. Overall, *H. pylori* infection is associated with a two- to sixfold increase in the risk of developing antral and body gastric cancer (Plate 6.2, facing p. 26). In 1994 the World Health Organization and the International Agency for Research on Cancer (IARC) classified *H. pylori* as a group I (definite) car-

There is a correlation between regional variations of gastric cancer and *H. pylori* infection

cinogen. *H. pylori* is now aligned with other biological carcinogens such as hepatitis B and C viruses.

Evidence supporting involvement of *H. pylori* in gastric cancer is epidemiological and is furnished by prolonged follow-up of subjects with and without *H. pylori* infection, diagnosed on the basis of positive serology performed on sera banked for other purposes. Development of atrophic gastritis and intestinal metaplasia, conditions recognised as part of the multi-step progression from normal mucosa to carcinoma, are significantly more common in subjects with *H. pylori* infection.

Atrophic gastritis and intestinal metaplasia are recognised stages in carcinoma evolution

Proposed mechanisms of carcinogenesis

It is not suggested that *H. pylori* is directly carcinogenic, but it sets the scene by causing gastritis and thus enables other luminal carcinogens to act on a mucosa damaged by the bacterium. A number of mechanisms have been proposed to account for the increased risk of developing stomach cancer in the presence of *H. pylori* infection. Studies have shown that *H. pylori* and the associated inflammatory response increases gastric epithelial proliferation, which is decreased after eradication of *H. pylori*. Furthermore, the neutrophil response induced by *H. pylori* can produce and release reactive oxygen free radicals, which can damage DNA. Vitamin C secretion by the gastric mucosa is decreased in the presence of *H. pylori* gastritis, and returns to normal after eradication of *H. pylori*. The lack of vitamin C in gastric juice may affect the capacity of the stomach to deal with the accumulation of carcinogenic nitroso compounds in gastric secretion.

The inflammatory response may lead to epithelial proliferation

Less than 1% of *H. pylori*-infected individuals will ever develop gastric cancer and, understandably, there is so far no evidence that the risk of gastric cancer is decreased by eradication of *H. pylori*. In clinical practice a patient who is aware of the cancer risk, or who comes from a 'cancer family', or who has first-degree relatives with gastric cancer, may ask for their *H. pylori* status to be determined and, if positive, to be treated. After appropriate counselling, eradication treatment should be offered in such circumstances.

There is no evidence that the risk of gastric cancer is reduced by *H. pylori* eradication

Gastric lymphoma and Ménétrier's disease

Gastric lymphoma of mucosa-associated lymphoid tissue (MALT)

Gastric lymphoma of MALT is a clonal B-cell malignancy that generally follows an indolent course and responds well to chemotherapy, although metastases or progression to large-cell lymphoma also occur. *H. pylori* infection has been associated with the acquisition of MALT and the subsequent development of malignant lymphoma. Dependence of early MALT lymphoma on growth stimulation by *H. pylori*-specific T lymphocytes was shown recently, suggesting that early tumours may be responsive to withdrawal of this stimulus. Indeed, eradication of *H. pylori* with antibiotic therapy has resulted in regression of low-grade B-cell gastric lymphoma of MALT type. Long-term follow-up studies of patients with gastric MALT lymphomas treated by eradication of *H. pylori* are needed before this treatment is recommended outside clinical trials.

H. pylori eradication has caused the regression of MALT lymphoma

Non-Hodgkin's lymphoma

Non-Hodgkin's lymphoma of the stomach is a rare disorder that accounts for only 3% of gastric malignancies. Epidemiological evidence suggests that *H. pylori* infection is associated with this disease, but no data are available on the effect of eradication of *H. pylori* in this condition.

Ménétrier's disease (hypertrophic gastropathy) is characterised by tortuous enlarged gastric folds and enteric protein loss leading to hypoalbuminaemia (Plate 6.3, facing p. 26). *H. pylori* infection is found in more than 90% of patients with this condition, and eradication of *H. pylori* has been reported to return the stomach and protein concentration to normal.

Over 90% of patients with Ménétrier's disease are colonised with *H. pylori*

Coronary heart disease

A case–control study recently reported that the crude odds ratio for risk of coronary heart disease associated with *H. pylori* seropositivity was 2.28. Age, socioeconomic status and ethnic group are all associated with *H. pylori* infection and with coronary heart disease, and so would be expected to confound this association. Thus, the odds ratio fell to 1.90 after adjustment for age, cardiovascular risk factors and socioeco-

The link between
coronary heart disease
and *H. pylori* infection is
surrounded by
controversy

nomic status. If this association does prove to be real, and not
the result of known or unidentified confounding factors, then
H. pylori infection may be an independent risk factor for coronary heart disease. The mechanism underlying the association between *H. pylori* and coronary heart disease may be
related to increased fibrinogen concentrations and blood clot-
ting activity, or elevated lipid peroxides in patients infected
with *H. pylori*. Further well-designed studies are needed to
confirm the interesting association between *H. pylori* and
coronary heart disease before any recommendations regarding
treatment can be made. It should be borne in mind that other
low-grade chronic infections, for example with *Chlamydia*,
have also been shown to be associated with coronary heart
disease.

Conclusion

H. pylori eradication is indicated in *H. pylori*-positive patients
with:
• non-NSAID DU (including complicated DU, for example,
with previous bleeding);
• benign, non-NSAID GU.
H. pylori eradication has no proven clinical benefit in patients
with:
• functional (non-ulcer) dyspepsia;
• ulcers associated with NSAIDs;
• asymptomatic individuals.

Further reading

Anonymous. *Helicobacter pylori* in peptic ulcer disease. NIH Consensus
Conference. *J Am Med Assoc* 1994; **272**: 65–9.
Bayerdörffer E, Rutter MM, Hatz R *et al*. Healing of protein-losing
hypertrophic gastropathy by eradication of *Helicobacter pylori*: is
Helicobacter pylori a pathogenic factor in Ménétrier's disease? *Gut*
1994; **35**: 701–4.
Forbes GM, Glaser ME, Cullen DJE *et al*. Duodenal ulcer treated with
Helicobacter pylori eradication: seven year follow-up. *Lancet* 1994;
334: 258–60.
Mendall MA, Goggin PM, Molineaux N *et al*. Relation of *Helicobacter
pylori* infection and coronary heart disease. *Br Heart J* 1994; **71**:
437–9.
Rauws BAJ, Tytgat GNJ. *Helicobacter pylori* in duodenal and gastric
ulcer disease. *Ballière's Clin Gastroenterol* 1995; **9**(3): 529–47.
The Eurogast Study Group. An international association between

Helicobacter pylori infection and gastric cancer. *Lancet* 1993; **341**: 1359–62.

Wotherspoon AC, Doglioni C, Diss TC *et al*. Regression of primary low-grade B-cell gastric lymphoma of mucosa-associated lymphoid tissue type after eradication of *Helicobacter pylori*. *Lancet* 1993; **342**: 575–7.

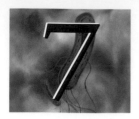

The development of a vaccine against *H. pylori*

Summary

- Vaccine has potentially 100% efficacy after a single dose without side effects.
- Vaccination may lead to life-long immunity.
- Vaccine may be preventative and therapeutic.
- Appropriate antigen must be identified; potential *H. pylori* antigens include CagA, VacA, urease and *Hp*cpn 10-1.

Background

H. pylori is probably the most common chronic bacterial infection in humans. It is the cause of the vast majority of peptic ulcer disease, and is strongly associated with an increased risk of gastric cancer and lymphoma, and possibly coronary heart disease. The bacterium can be successfully eradicated from the foregut by a 1-week combination of three or four drugs in around 90% of subjects, but the occurrence of resistance to antibiotics, the possibility of re-infection and the cost implications for developing countries, makes this therapeutic approach less attractive in the long term. Vaccination is a more promising preventative and therapeutic approach, whereby a single dose of an oral vaccine may eradicate current infection with *H. pylori* and lead to life-long immunity from re-infection with the organism.

Cost implications of eradication make vaccination an attractive possibility

H. pylori is a remarkably well-adapted human pathogen that colonises its host for life, despite strong systemic and mucosal immune responses. Indeed, *H. pylori* is able to survive in gastric mucus or attached to gastric epithelial cells despite being surrounded by phagocytes and cytokine-secreting lymphocytes. Thus, activation of the immune system against colonisation of the foregut by *H. pylori* appears insufficient to eliminate the infection. It is these properties of the bacterium that make the development of a therapeutic vaccine against *H. pylori* infection so challenging. Furthermore, as there are no

H. pylori's ability to survive attack by its host's immune system makes it a challenging candidate for a vaccine

natural animal reservoirs of *H. pylori*, animal models of *Helicobacter* infection have had to be developed.

Vaccine antigens

VacA and CagA

H. pylori strains can be classified as type I and type II (see Chapter 3). Type I strains make up about 65% of the total and produce VacA (vacuolating cytotoxin) and CagA (cytotoxin-associated protein). Type II bacteria account for about 20% of the remainder, and produce neither VacA toxin nor CagA protein. About 15% of isolates fall in between these classifications. Most patients with duodenal ulcer disease are colonised by a type I strain of *H. pylori*, and this makes the presence of VacA and/or CagA an interesting candidate for vaccination. Indeed, oral immunisation with purified VacA plus an adjuvant to stimulate the immune system (*Escherichia coli* heat-labile toxin in this case) has recently been shown to protect against *H. pylori* colonisation in a mouse model.

Vaccination against type I with VacA looks promising in a mouse model

Urease

Urease production has been detected in all clinical strains of *H. pylori*. This nickel-containing enzyme has two subunits: A and B. Oral administration of *H. pylori* urease, or its subunits, plus cholera toxin as adjuvant, has been reported to prevent infection by *H. pylori* in the mouse.

*Hp*cpn 10-1

The *H. pylori* genome contains a *Hp*cpn10 gene which encodes for *Hp*cpn10 (13 kDa)—termed chaperonin (cpn) 10-1. Chaperonins promote the folding and assembly of oligomeric proteins to minimise gastric acid-induced denaturing effects on protein tertiary structure. *Hp*cpn 10-1 has nickel-binding activities and is responsible for the activation of the urease enzyme. The DNA region encoding the A domain of *Hp*cpn 10-1 was reported to be highly conserved in all clinical isolates of *H. pylori*, whereas the B domain displayed some polymorphism; thus, *Hp*cpn 10-1 could turn out to be a good candidate for a protective antigen.

Chaperonins may prove to be protective antigens

Adjuvant

The mucosal adjuvants used in the animal models, such as cholera or *E. coli* toxin, may be highly toxic or even life-threatening in humans. Recently, a promising approach was reported using genetically detoxified mutants of *E. coli* toxin that maintain their adjuvant activity.

Prevention and cure?

Pre-existing infection may also be eradicated with a vaccine

The observation that oral immunisation with *Helicobacter* antigens can induce protection against infection in mouse models is an important landmark in the development of preventative strategies in humans. The next step was to establish whether the immunisation procedure could eradicate an established infection from the foregut. Recent reports have indicated that oral treatment with recombinant *H. pylori* urease in mice leads to protection against a challenge with *H. felis*. These preliminary data raise the possibility that oral immunisation with *H. pylori* antigens may lead to long-lasting protection from infection and, furthermore, eradicate pre-existing infection with *H. pylori*.

The future

The vaccine approach to *H. pylori* infection in humans is preferable to the use of triple or quadruple drug treatment regimens for several reasons.

A *H. pylori* vaccine would have numerous advantages over eradication therapy

1 Antibiotics are associated with side effects, some of which are serious (pseudomembranous colitis), require multiple doses and need to be taken for at least 7 days. By contrast, an oral vaccine may need to be given once only, and without serious side effects.

2 Resistance to antibiotics is an increasing problem and may lead to failure in some subjects despite repeated treatment courses. Vaccination with an antigen that is present in all clinical isolates, such as urease, an essential virulence factor of *H. pylori*, should overcome all strains of *H. pylori*.

3 Eradication success or failure with current treatment regimens is dependent upon patient compliance. No such problem would occur with a vaccine.

4 Eradication treatment may cure current infection with *H. pylori*, whereas vaccination not only eradicates *H. pylori*, but should prevent re-infection.

Further reading

Lee A. Animal models and vaccine development. *Baillière's Clin Gastroenterol* 1995; **9**(3): 615–32.

Index